P9-DDW-579

THE CANCER
SURVIVOR'S
GUIDE

FOODS THAT HELP YOU FIGHT BACK

Neal D. Barnard, MD

Jennifer K. Reilly, RD

HEALTHY LIVING PUBLICATIONS
Summertown, TN 38483

Library of Congress Cataloging-in-Publication Data

Barnard, Neal D., 1953-
   The cancer survivor's guide : foods that help you fight back / Neal D.
Barnard, Jennifer K. Reilly.
       p. cm.
   Includes bibliographical references.
   ISBN 978-1-57067-225-5
   1. Cancer—Nutritional aspects.   2. Cancer—Prevention.   3. Cancer—Diet
therapy. I. Reilly, Jennifer K. II. Title.

   RC268.45.B37 2008
   616.99'40654—dc22

                                          2008041092

© 2008 The Cancer Project

Cover and interior design: *Aerocraft Charter Art Service*

All rights reserved. No portion of this book may be reproduced by any means whatsoever, except for brief quotations in reviews, without written permission from the publisher.

Printed in Canada

Healthy Living Publications, a division of
Book Publishing Company
P.O. Box 99
Summertown, TN 38483
888-260-8458
www.bookpubco.com

ISBN: 978-1-57067-225-5

17 16 15 14 13 12 11 10   4 5 6 7 8 9 10 11

Book Publishing Co. is a member of Green Press Initiative. We chose to print this title on paper with postconsumer recycled content, processed without chlorine, which saved the following natural resources:

103 trees

7,593 pounds of solid waste

88,387 gallons of water

23,399 pounds of greenhouse gases

119 million BTU of total energy

For more information, visit
www.greenpressinitiative.org.

Paper calculations from Environmental Defense Paper Calculator, www.edf.org/papercalculator

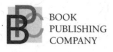

CONTENTS

A Note to the Reader   v

Introduction
How Foods Fight Cancer   vii

1 **Fueling Up on Low-Fat Foods**   1

2 **Favoring Fiber**   9

3 **Discovering Dairy Alternatives**   17

4 **Replacing Meat**   25

5 **Cancer-Fighting Compounds and Immune-Boosting Foods**   29

6 **Maintaining a Healthy Weight**   43

7 **Foods and Breast Cancer Survival**   47

8 **Foods and Prostate Cancer Survival**   53

9 **Planning Health-Promoting Meals**   57

10 **Questions and Answers**
ABOUT FOODS AND CANCER PREVENTION AND SURVIVAL   69

11 **Nutrition Basics**   85

12 RECIPES   89

Breakfast Ideas   90

Smoothies   99

Appetizers   105

Soups, Stews, and Chilis   120

Salads and Salad Dressings   134

Sauces and Gravies   154

Basic Grains   158

Grain Side Dishes   164

Vegetable Side Dishes   171

Main Dishes   185

Sandwiches, Burgers, and Wraps   202

Desserts   212

Recipe Contributors   225
References   227
Additional Resources   233
Index   235

A NOTE TO THE READER

The Cancer Survivor's Guide: Foods that Help You Fight Back was written by Neal D. Barnard, MD, with the help of Jennifer K. Reilly, RD. The recipes were developed by Jennifer Raymond, MS, RD, with additional contributions and assistance from Amy Lanou, PhD, Brie Turner-McGrievy, MS, RD, Jennifer Reilly, RD, Stephanie Beine, RD, Evelisse Capo, and Brandi Redo. This handbook was created to accompany The Cancer Project's "Food for Life Nutrition and Cooking Class Series for Cancer Prevention and Survival." However, it is sufficiently detailed to be used on its own and will give you important insights into food's role in cancer prevention and cancer survival.

Our goal is to provide you with information about food and health. However, neither this book nor any other can take the place of individualized medical care or advice. All cancer treatments, including dietary changes, must take into account your needs as an individual. In addition, if you are overweight, have any health problem, or are on medication, you should consult with your doctor before making any modifications to your diet or exercise routines, and you should follow your doctor's recommendations, which will be based on your personal needs.

There are many situations in which a dietary change can alter your need for medications. For example, individuals with diabetes, high blood pressure, or high cholesterol levels often need less medication when they improve their diets. You should be sure to work with your physician to adjust your regimen as needed.

The science of nutrition grows gradually as time goes on, so we encourage you to consult other sources of information, including the Additional Resources section on page 227.

With any dietary change, it is important to ensure complete nutrition. Be sure to include a source of vitamin B_{12} in your routine, which could include any common multivitamin, fortified soymilk or cereals, or a vitamin B_{12} supplement of five micrograms or more per day.

We wish you the very best of health.

How Foods Fight Cancer

F or many years, researchers have been investigating how food choices can help prevent cancer and, when cancer has been diagnosed, how these choices can improve survival. While their work is by no means finished, what is already known is nothing short of dramatic. Certain diet patterns seem to have a major effect, helping people diagnosed with cancer to live longer, healthier lives. Other diet choices are risky propositions, increasing the toll cancer takes.

Our goal is to translate scientific findings into simple, practical steps you can use in your own kitchen, at the grocery store, at restaurants—anywhere you're thinking about what to eat. We'll divide this information into eight chapters and include key scientific information, meal-planning tips, and suggested steps you can take at home. We will also list recipes that illustrate the key points in each chapter. Some recipes embody more than one nutritional advantage, so we'll list especially good ones in more than one chapter. All the recipes (and more) are included in this book.

Before we begin, one note of caution: As we explore the role of food in cancer, some people might feel a bit uneasy. If foods can affect cancer risk, they ask, does that mean I am somehow to blame for my illness? Did the foods I ate as a child cause this problem? Is our culture causing these problems?

It is natural that concerns like these will cross our minds. However, let us encourage you to set blame aside. The fact is, some people do their very best to follow health-promoting lifestyles and still develop cancer. And you may have known people who smoke, drink heavily, and eat with abandon and yet manage to live to a ripe old age. Unfortunately, it is easy to get cancer, and we cannot predict with certainty who will be affected by it and who will not. So let's focus not on blame but on what foods can do for you. As Jack Nicklaus said, "You can spend all day trying to figure out why you hit your ball into the woods—or you can just go in and get it out."

Certain diet patterns seem to have a major effect, helping people diagnosed with cancer to live longer, healthier lives.

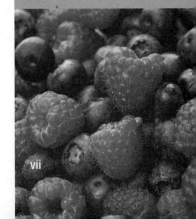

Research into food's role in cancer survival grew from studies looking at the causes of the illness. As researchers compared the diets of people who developed cancer and those of people who remained healthy, they found many factors that do indeed influence cancer risk. They also had an opportunity to look forward to see how various eating patterns affect survival.

High Fiber, Low Fat

It turns out that many foods that help prevent cancer in the first place also seem to help us beat the disease when it has struck. Among the most important themes to emerge from research has been that foods influence the hormones that fuel cancer growth. For example, diets high in fiber and low in fat tend to reduce the amount of estrogens (female sex hormones) circulating in the bloodstream. This taming of estrogens seems to reduce the likelihood that cancer cells will multiply or spread.

Fiber is also important in preventing colon cancer, as it helps move food waste out of the body. And fiber may even help the immune system function properly. Building your diet from fiber-rich plant foods is important for cancer prevention and survival as well as overall health. In chapters 1 and 2, you'll learn about building low-fat, fiber-rich foods into your routine.

Reasons to Avoid Dairy Products

Typical dairy products (milk, cheese, yogurt, and so forth) are loaded with fat and cholesterol, and researchers are discovering that dairy products appear to play an important role in cancer risk. Harvard researchers in the Physicians' Health Study and the Health Professionals Follow-Up Study found that men who frequently consume dairy products had a higher prostate cancer risk. Possible reasons for this connection include dairy products' tendency to boost *insulin-like growth factor 1* (IGF-1) production in the body and the high calcium content of dairy products, which decreases vitamin D activation. Breast cancer and ovarian cancer risk have also been examined for their links to dairy consumption. Happily, soymilk, rice milk, nondairy yogurt, and other dairy alternatives make the switch easy, as you'll learn in chapter 3.

Avoiding Meat

Numerous research studies have shown that cancer is more common in populations consuming diets rich in fatty foods, particularly meat, and much less common in countries with diets rich in grains, vegetables, and fruits. Evidence suggests that this is partly due to the high-fat and fiber-free characteristics of meat compared to plant foods. In addition, because meats are cooked, cancer-causing chemicals called *heterocyclic amines* tend to form within the meat tissue. The longer and hotter meat is cooked, the more these compounds form. In chapter 4, you will learn more about how meat is linked to cancer risk, and also about vegetarian sources of protein, which are low in fat, high in fiber, and loaded with cancer-fighting nutrients.

Cancer Fighters in Plant Foods and Immune-Boosting Foods

Antioxidants are powerful cancer fighters mainly found in vegetables and fruits. They assist in halting free radical damage, which can otherwise lead to cancer development. Chapter 5 will look in some detail at which vegetables and fruits are high in which protective compounds. The key message is *to be generous with a variety of vegetables and fruits* as you plan your menu. Studies have amply demonstrated the ability of diets rich in vegetables and fruits to reduce the likelihood that cancer will develop in the first place. Studies have also suggested that cancer survivors who consume more vegetables and fruits do indeed live longer, cancer-free lives.

Chapter 5 will also explore the immune system's role in fighting cancer. Beta-carotene, vitamin C, and zinc can help the immune system recognize and destroy cancer cells. In contrast, foods rich in fat and cholesterol can interfere with immunity. Studies have shown that vegetarians have approximately double the natural killer cell activity (natural killer cells engulf and destroy cancer cells) compared to nonvegetarians.

Maintaining a Healthy Weight

Healthy weight control is essential for warding off a variety of chronic diseases, and studies have shown that slimmer people are less likely to develop cancer. In addition, trimming excess weight may also improve survival after cancer has been diagnosed. Chapter 6 covers the basics of healthy weight control.

Jump Right In

Many parts of the diet can help us stay healthy or regain health when we're dealing with illness. Vegetables, fruits, beans, whole grains, and many other foods have been under study for some time. While we do not have all the answers, we have more than enough information to get started with more healthful ways of eating.

As we begin, let us encourage you not to simply dabble with dietary changes. If you or a loved one have been diagnosed with a major illness, it is time to take full advantage of what your diet can do for you. Much as we might like to pretend that small dietary changes help, the fact is that trimming a little fat here and adding a piece of fruit there does very little.

That has been proven true in studies using diet to control cholesterol, diabetes, hypertension, osteoporosis, weight problems, and many other conditions. So we will not sell you short with half-baked dietary suggestions. Rather, we will encourage you to jump in and take full advantage of what these foods can offer. Chances are, you will love where you're headed. An exploration of healthful eating may not only bring you better health; it may also lead to new and interesting tastes, exotic restaurants, and some of the most remarkable aisles in the grocery store.

Yes, you'll have some challenges along the way. A new recipe might turn out to be stunning, or it could also be a dud. Don't worry. That's what experimenting is all about. As you get to know what works for you, you'll discover a new world of nutritious, powerful foods and delicious tastes, and an entirely new way of thinking about food and health.

To Do This Week

THE 3-3-3 WAY TO REVAMP YOUR DIET

If you're going to stick with health-promoting foods for three weeks—or for the rest of your life—you don't have to be a gourmet chef. If you think about it, most of us choose our dinner on any given night from only about eight or nine different favorite meals that make up our culinary repertoires. So, when you're revamping your menu, all you need are eight or nine *healthful* meals that you like. Once you've found them, you've got everything you need.

Try this: Jot down on a piece of paper the names of three meals you already like that contain no animal products and are reasonably low in fat. For example, you might choose pasta with a marinara sauce, a bean and rice burrito filled with grilled vegetables, a garden salad with kidney beans and low-fat Italian dressing, a portobello mushroom sandwich with roasted red peppers, or veggie chili with crackers.

Next, write down three more meals you like that could be easily modified to eliminate animal products and added fat. Examples might include a vegetable stew instead of the beefy variety, a stir-fry with vegetables instead of chicken, a taco salad made with beans and chunky vegetables instead of meat, or a veggie burger instead of the usual meat patty.

Finally, write down three meals that are new to you that you'd like to try. Take a look at the recipes on pages 186 to 211 for ideas and pick out three that appeal to you.

Now, if you have done this exercise thoughtfully, you've found nine meals that are likely to work for you, and you have just solved your problem. There are many other great foods to try, of course, but you are off to a tremendous start.

Fueling Up on Low-Fat Foods

Many teams of researchers have studied the health of various populations around the world, hoping to tease out the causes of cancer and ways to prevent it. In one study after another, they have found that people following plant-based diets tend to have strikingly low cancer rates. In rural Asia and Africa, for example, traditional diets are based on rice or other grains, starchy vegetables, fruits, and beans, and people eating these diets generally avoid the disease. If cancer does strike, they also seem to have better survival rates.

When these populations trade their traditional diets for a menu based on Western foods—either because they have migrated or because fast-food restaurants and other Western food purveyors have come to them—their cancer rates promptly change. In Japan, dramatic diet changes began after World War II. Traditional rice dishes were gradually replaced with hamburgers. Dairy products, which had been almost unknown in Japan, became popular. Carbohydrate intake fell, and fat consumption soared. Soon, cancer rates began to rise, as did the toll of obesity, heart problems, and other diseases.

Although many factors may be at work here, let us focus first on one key biological fact: High-fat, low-fiber foods boost the hormones that promote cancer. Specifically, diets rich in meat, dairy products, fried foods, and even vegetable oils cause a woman's body to make more estrogen. The term "estrogen" actually refers to a group of hormones, including estradiol, estrone, and others. For simplicity, they will be referred to here as "estrogen." In turn, that extra estrogen increases cancer risk in the breast and other organs that are sensitive to female sex hormones.

To see why this matters, think for a moment about estrogen's role in the body. In simple terms, estrogen makes things grow. As an adolescent girl develops a mature figure, she experiences estrogen's ability to stimulate the growth of breast tissue. The hormone also thickens the lining of the uterus every month as a woman's body prepares for the possibility of pregnancy.

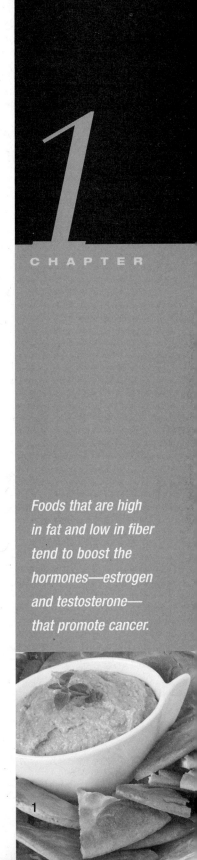

Foods that are high in fat and low in fiber tend to boost the hormones—estrogen and testosterone— that promote cancer.

Estrogen not only makes normal tissues grow; it can also make cancer cells grow. Although researchers have long known that estrogens encourage the growth of cancer cells once they form, evidence also suggests that they can also spark the very first step in cancer development: the transformation of healthy cells into cancer cells. Specifically, enzymes in the body alter estrogens to produce other molecules that can damage DNA, leading to cancer. When researchers add a bit of estrogen to breast cancer cells in a test tube, they multiply rapidly.[1] In fact, one of the main goals of breast cancer treatment is to reduce estrogen's effects (using drugs, such as tamoxifen, that block estrogen's activity).

Here is where diet comes in. Foods influence estrogen's effect, too—to a striking degree. When a woman begins a low-fat, high-fiber diet, the amount of estrogen in her blood drops almost immediately. In a matter of weeks, the amount in her bloodstream drops by 15–50 percent.[2,3] She will still have more than enough estrogen for fertility, but she will nonetheless have less estrogen than before. From the standpoint of cancer prevention, that's a good thing. It means there will be less stimulus for cancer cell growth.

A 2003 study published in the *Journal of the National Cancer Institute* found that when girls aged eight to ten reduced the amount of fat in their diets—even very slightly—their estrogen levels were held at a lower and safer level during the next several years. When the girls increased their intake of vegetables, fruits, grains, and beans, and reduced their intake of animal-derived foods, the amount of estradiol (a principal estrogen) in their blood dropped by 30 percent compared to a group of girls who did not change their diets.[4]

The same phenomenon occurs in men. Men have estrogen in their blood, too—although much less than women have—and cancer researchers have long suspected that both estrogen and testosterone (the "male hormone") play roles in prostate cancer risk. But as men cut the fat and increase fiber in their diets, the amounts of both estrogen and testosterone tend to fall. Don't worry—this change does not make a man any less masculine. But it may well reduce the hormonal stimulus for prostate cancer growth.

Because of these and related findings, many researchers have suggested that steering clear of meat, dairy products, fried foods, and other fatty fare may reduce cancer risk. However, it is important to understand that, in order to reduce cancer risk or effectively alter its course, dietary changes have to be significant. Studies have shown that modest changes in diet do little or nothing. For example, in the Women's Health Initiative study, nearly 25,000 women in the intervention group were instructed to consume a low-fat diet (aiming for no more than 20 percent of calories from fat) for eight years.[5] However, the inclusion of naturally high-fat meat and dairy products in the diet made it difficult for participants to meet the moderately low-fat requirement and show any signs of cancer risk reduction. By the end of the study, these women were averaging 29 percent of calories from fat, compared to the control group, which averaged 35 percent of calories from fat. This modest difference resulted in only small changes in breast cancer risk reduction.

There were some bright spots in the study. Risk of progesterone-negative tumors fell by 30 percent. And those women who made the greatest reductions in fat intake had a more significant drop in overall risk, up to 20 percent. Large studies of American women have shown that moderate variations in fat intake made no difference in their breast cancer risk. The best evidence suggests that, to be effective, dietary changes have to be sizable.

Nonetheless, research bears out a major effect of diet, not only on cancer prevention, but also on cancer survival. Breast cancer patients who follow lower-fat diets do tend to live substantially longer. Researchers at the State University of New York in Buffalo tracked the diets of 953 women who had been diagnosed with breast cancer. They then followed them to see who did well and who did not. The results were striking. The risk of dying at any point in time increased by 40 percent for every 1,000 grams of fat the women consumed per month.[6]

> The risk of dying at any point in time increased by 40 percent for every 1,000 grams of fat the women consumed per month.

Let's see what this means in practical terms: If you were to add up all the fat in a typical American diet over the course of a month and compare it to the amount of fat in a low-fat, pure vegetarian diet, the two would differ by approximate 1,500 grams of fat each month. If the study's findings hold, that would correspond to a 60 percent increased risk of dying at any point in time for patients following a typical American diet.

Several other studies have found much the same thing: Women with breast cancer who eat fattier foods—meats, dairy products, and fried foods—have greater rates of cancer recurrence and succumb more frequently than do those whose diets are based on the lower-fat choices—vegetables, fruits, whole grains, and beans.[7] Frightening as this sort of finding may be, it shows us a path toward reducing the need for further treatment and improves the odds of living a life free of the tolls cancer can take.

Similar findings have emerged about prostate cancer. Men on more health-promoting diets—that is, diets rich in vegetables, fruits, and other low-fat foods from plant sources—are less likely to develop cancer in the first place and, if cancer does strike, are more likely to survive it.[8,9]

Chicken Is Not a Vegetable

Many people try to trim fat from their diets by switching from beef to chicken. Unfortunately, chicken has nearly as much fat as beef. As you'll see in table 1, the leanest beef is about 28 percent fat (as a percentage of calories). The leanest chicken—skinless breast meat, prepared without added fat—is not much better at about 24 percent. Fish vary, with some lower

TABLE 1 Fat in foods

FOOD	PERCENTAGE OF CALORIES FROM FAT
salmon, Atlantic, wild	40
beef, round bottom, lean	28
chicken, white meat, skinless	24
tuna, white	21
broccoli, raw	10
rice, brown	7
beans, navy	4
lentils	3
apple	3
orange	2

Source: U.S. Department of Agriculture, Agricultural Research Service. 2007. USDA National Nutrient Database for Standard Reference, Release 20. Nutrient Data Laboratory Home Page, *www.nal.usda.gov/fnic/foodcomp.*

than chicken and some higher, but the truly low-fat foods are in a class by themselves: Beans, vegetables, fruits, and whole grains are all very low in fat and, as we'll see in later chapters, high in vitamins, minerals, and healthful fiber.

If you or your loved ones are trying to eliminate fat from your diet, switching from beef to chicken does not bring you very far. On the other hand, building your menu from whole grains, beans, vegetables, and fruits is a powerful way to trim the fat.

We'll conclude this section with the results from a surprising experiment conducted at the University of California at Los Angeles. Researchers drew blood samples from a group of men who had been following a low-fat diet and exercising regularly for several years. They also drew blood samples from overweight men who were not following any diet or exercise program. They then added portions of each man's blood serum to test tubes containing standardized prostate cancer cells. It turned out that serum from men on the low-fat diet and exercise program slowed cancer cell growth by 49 percent compared to serum from the other men. The changes in diet and exercise had caused the amount of testosterone, estrogen, and other components in the blood to change so dramatically that the effect on cancer cells was obvious right in the test tube.[10]

The effect occurs quickly. The research team found cancer-inhibiting power within as little as eleven days after beginning a low-fat diet and exercise regimen.[11]

Building your menu from whole grains, beans, vegetables, and fruits is a powerful way to trim the fat.

TABLE 2 The New Four Food Groups

FOOD GROUP	SUGGESTED DAILY SERVINGS	SERVING SIZE
fruits	3 or more	½ cup; 1 whole
legumes (beans, peas, and lentils)	3 or more	½ cup cooked beans; ¼ cup bean spread; 1 cup nondairy milk; 3 ounces tofu, tempeh, seitan, or meat alternative
vegetables	4 or more	1 cup raw; ½ cup cooked
whole grains	6 or more	½ cup cooked; ¾–1 cup dry cereal; 1 slice of bread; ½ tortilla; a bagel is 4 servings

Cutting down on fat is an important first step in preventing cancer and in surviving it if it has been diagnosed. So how do we go about it? The easiest way is to build your meals from foods that are naturally low in fat and to use cooking methods that don't require you to add fats or oils.

Meal Planning: The New Four Food Groups

The easiest and perhaps most useful guide to basic nutrition is called the New Four Food Groups, introduced by the Physicians Committee for Responsible Medicine in 1991. Let us briefly review the guidelines; then, we will see how to turn them into actual meals.

The New Four Food Groups are vegetables, legumes, fruits, and whole grains. The idea is to build your diet by choosing a variety from each of these groups. Table 2 provides the suggested number of daily servings from each group (for more details and serving sizes, see table 17, page 59). Add any common multiple vitamin to ensure adequate intake of vitamin B_{12}.

The serving numbers listed in table 2 are just suggestions to get you started. Feel free to vary your proportions as you like. For example, one way of using the New Four Food Groups follows a traditional Asian pattern, favoring grains, such as rice or noodles, with smaller amounts of vegetables and bean dishes, and reserving fruit for dessert. However, it is just as acceptable to emphasize more vegetables and fewer grain products. Some people who gravitate toward raw foods will increase fruits. You can get complete and healthful nutrition using essentially any pattern that includes each of the four groups.

For optimal nutrition, you will want to avoid meat (red meat, poultry, and fish), dairy products, eggs, added oils, and high-fat foods (potato chips, french fries, onion rings, olives, and so forth). Limit nuts and nut butters, seeds, and avocados. Steer clear of fried foods and any oily or fatty toppings, such as margarine or typical salad dressings (nonfat dressings are fine). Avoiding fatty foods helps your taste buds to reduce their preference for greasy tastes. When you select breads, cereals, or other grain products, favor those that retain their natural fiber (for example, choose brown rice rather than white rice).

So how does all this translate into actual meals? The foods you'll now focus on are really not so different from what you already eat. Breakfast might be a big bowl of old-fashioned oatmeal with cinnamon and raisins (but skip the milk). If you like, add some cantaloupe or whole-grain toast. Lunch might be a bowl of split pea soup with a whole-grain roll or a plate of hummus, fresh veggies, and pita bread. Dinner could be minestrone followed by angel hair pasta with marinara sauce, or perhaps an autumn stew of vegetables, beans, and hearty grains.

Recommended Recipes

- Gingered Melon (page 218)
- Roasted Red Pepper Hummus (page 113)
- Sweet-and-Sour Stir-Fry (page 200)
- Toasted Grains (see page 163)

To Do This Week

CHECK YOUR DIET WITH A THREE-DAY DIETARY RECORD

You can get a good idea of the healthfulness of your overall diet with a three-day dietary record. This is the same diet-tracking tool that researchers use in clinical studies. It not only lets you see exactly what you're eating now, it also helps you see how to improve your diet over time. If, for example, you're getting a little too much fat or too little fiber, you'll spot it right away and can fix the problem.

To do your record, you simply take a sheet of paper and note down everything you eat or drink (except water) for three days, including two weekdays and one weekend day (most of us eat a bit differently on weekends compared to weekdays).

Using the Diet Record form on page 8 (photocopy it as many times as needed), jot down each food, condiment, or beverage on a separate line. For example, if you had a salad made of lettuce, tomatoes, chickpeas, and dressing, use four lines, one for each ingredient. Or if you had a peanut butter and jelly sandwich, along with a cola, use four lines so you can separate out each part of the meal—bread, peanut butter, jelly, and the drink.

Write down everything you eat, including snacks and condiments. The only item to omit from the list is your water consumption. Record the amount of each food as accurately as you can. You can either weigh each item using a food scale (available in stores that sell kitchenware) or measure or estimate its volume (for example, one cup of orange juice, or perhaps a small, medium, or large apple).

Record your foods as you go so you don't forget. If it is more convenient, you can keep notes in a small notebook and transfer them to the Diet Record form later. Be thorough.

If you like, you can get a detailed nutrient analysis of your diet. Just be sure to fill in the quantities carefully and use a food scale. A dietitian can analyze the record for you, or you can simply log in to a nutrient-analysis Web site, such as the University of Illinois Food Science and Human Nutrition Department's site *www.nat.uiuc.edu/mainnat.html*, *www.dietsite.com*, or *www.NutritionMD.org*. Please note that while the nutrient analyses on these sites are generally accurate, some of their nutrition guidelines are not necessarily optimal. Many commonly used guidelines allow too much fat and cholesterol. Here is a better set of goals: For an adult consuming 2,000 calories per day, a good fat-intake goal is about 25–35 grams each day. This works out to about 10–15 percent of calories. Cholesterol intake should be zero. Your protein intake should be roughly 50 grams per day. Resist the temptation to push protein intake too high.

Diet Record

Make as many copies of this page as you need. Record only one ingredient per line.　　　DATE: _____

TIME OF DAY	FOOD	AMOUNT	COOKING METHOD

Favoring Fiber

As you recall from the previous chapter, dietary changes can help reduce the amount of estrogen and testosterone in the bloodstream. Fiber is a key part of this. Fiber has other important benefits, too, as we'll see in this chapter.

"Fiber" is another word for plant roughage—the part of beans, grains, vegetables, and fruits that resists digestion. Fiber helps to keep us regular by moving the intestinal contents along. But it has other equally important roles. It helps us rid ourselves of all manner of chemicals—including hormones—that our bodies are anxious to eliminate.

This "waste disposal" system starts in your liver, which continuously filters your blood. As blood passes through the liver's network of tiny capillaries, liver cells remove toxins, cholesterol, medications, waste hormones, and whatever else your body figures it is better off without. These undesirables are then sent from the liver into a small tube called the bile duct, which leads to your intestinal tract. There, fiber soaks up these chemicals and carries them out with the wastes.

Now, there is plenty of fiber in vegetables, fruits, beans, and whole grains. So if these foods are a big part of your diet, your "waste disposal" system works pretty well. The liver pulls hormones out of the bloodstream, they slide down the bile duct, fiber picks them up, and out they go.

But what happens if your lunch consisted of a chicken breast and a cup of yogurt? These products don't come from plants—and that means they have no fiber at all. Not a speck. So when your liver sends hormones or other chemicals into the intestinal tract, there is nothing for them to attach to. They end up being reabsorbed back into your bloodstream, and the whole process starts over again. This endless cycle—hormones passing from the bloodstream, through the liver, into the intestinal tract, and, unfortunately, back into the bloodstream—is called enterohepatic circulation. It keeps hormones circulating for longer than they should. Fiber stops this cycle by carrying hormones out once and for all.

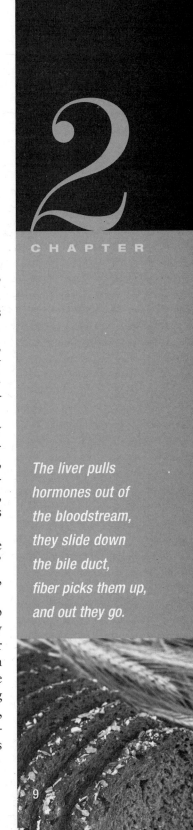

The liver pulls hormones out of the bloodstream, they slide down the bile duct, fiber picks them up, and out they go.

9

Fiber versus Colon Cancer

Fiber has another function you should know about. It may reduce your risk of colon cancer. Fiber moves intestinal contents along, so that whatever carcinogens (that is, cancer-causing chemicals) may be lurking in your waste products are escorted out of the body more quickly.

Carcinogens don't just come from factory waste and air pollution; they are sometimes present in foods. For example, when chicken, fish, or red meat is cooked at a high temperature, cancer-causing chemicals called heterocyclic amines tend to form as the protein molecules and other parts of muscle tissue are distorted by the intense heat. Needless to say, that is another good reason to avoid these products. However, the bile your body produces to digest fats can also encourage the production of carcinogens. A high-fiber diet helps move these compounds out of your body.

Aim for 40 Grams per Day

So, where do you find the fiber you need? Animal products don't have any. That goes for red meat, poultry, fish, eggs, and dairy products, which is why people who center their diets on these foods often struggle with constipation. On the other hand, plant products in their natural state have quite a lot of fiber, which is why vegetarians rarely have any need for laxatives. The first key to building a high-fiber diet is to eat plenty of vegetables, fruits, beans, and whole grains and to avoid animal products.

But a meaty diet is not the only wrong turn you can take. Let's say that for breakfast you had a choice between old-fashioned oatmeal with whole-grain toast on the one hand, and a bagel and jam on the other. The first breakfast is loaded with fiber, but a bagel has very little. It is made from white flour—that is, wheat flour whose fiber has been removed in the refining process. Refining makes it soft and white, but it leaves flour almost devoid of fiber.

If you choose whole-grain bread instead of white bread, you'll get much more fiber. The same is true for brown rice, which retains the grain's tan-colored outer layer, as opposed to white rice, which has lost this high-fiber layer in the refining process.

Generally speaking, the most fiber-rich foods are beans and vegetables, followed by fruits and whole grains. Yes, breakfast cereals and other grain products advertise their high-fiber content. But you'll find surprisingly large amounts of it in simple bean and vegetable dishes. Fiber comes in two forms:

Soluble fiber is the kind that dissolves in water, in the way that oatmeal, for example, gets creamy as it cooks. There is also plenty of soluble fiber in beans, barley, and several other foods. Soluble fiber is especially known for its ability to control cholesterol levels.

Insoluble fiber, which is found in vegetables, fruit, wheat, rice, and many other grains, is visibly different. Rice and wheat grains don't get "gooey" the way oatmeal does. Insoluble fiber is especially helpful for keeping the intestinal contents moving along and fighting constipation.

From the standpoint of cancer prevention, you'll want to get both kinds. If your diet is rich in beans, vegetables, fruits, and whole grains, you'll get plenty of healthful fiber. An average American gets only 10–15 grams of fiber per day. Health authorities would like to see that number rise significantly. A sensible and easily reached goal is 40 grams per day. Having said that, you may wish to reach this goal gradually, rather than in one jump. It may take a few weeks for your digestive tract to get used to the change.

Whole grains, such as brown rice and old-fashioned oatmeal, are pretty easy to digest. You'll find that cruciferous vegetables, such as broccoli, cabbage, and cauliflower, are easier to digest if they are cooked until soft. If beans cause gas for you, start with smaller quantities, be sure they are well cooked, and try different varieties.

Quick Fiber Check

The Quick Fiber Check is a handy little tool. Using its simple scoring concept, which takes only a minute or two to learn, you'll be able to estimate the fiber content of virtually everything in the grocery store and calculate your own fiber intake.

To check your meals, write down everything you eat or drink for one full day on the form that follows. Next to each food, jot in its fiber score, using the following guide:

- **Beans:** For each half-cup serving of beans or lentils or any food that includes about this amount of beans or lentils as an ingredient, mark 7. That is the number of grams of fiber in a serving. One cup of soymilk or one-half cup of tofu rates 3.
- **Vegetables:** For each one-cup serving of vegetables, mark 4. An exception is lettuce, for which one cup scores 2. A potato with skin scores 4; without the skin, it scores 2.
- **Fruit:** For each medium piece of fruit (for example, an apple, orange, or banana, one cup of applesauce, or a banana smoothie), mark 3. For one cup of juice, mark 1.
- **Grains:** For each piece of white bread, bagel, or equivalent, score 1. Whole-grain breads score 2. One cup of cooked pasta scores 2. One cup of rice scores 1 for white and 3 for brown. One cup of cooked oatmeal scores 4. Score 3 for typical ready-to-eat cereals, 1 for highly processed and colored cereals, and 8 for bran, or check the package information for grams of fiber.
- **Meat, poultry, or fish:** Score 0. Animal products do not contain fiber.
- **Eggs or dairy products:** Score 0.
- **Sodas, water:** Score 0.

Quick Fiber Check

FOOD (one food or ingredient per line)	FIBER SCORE

TOTAL FIBER SCORE: _____

Interpreting Your Quick Fiber Check Score

Less than 20: You need more fiber in your diet. As it is, your appetite will be hard to control, and you may have occasional constipation. Boosting fiber will help tame your appetite and can cut your risk of many health problems.

20–39: You are doing better than most people in Western countries, but as you bring more fiber into your diet, you will find that it makes foods more satisfying and cuts your calorie intake a bit.

40 or more: Congratulations! You have plenty of healthful fiber in your diet. It tames your appetite and helps keep you healthy. Fiber also reduces your risk of cancer, heart disease, diabetes, and digestive problems.

High-Fiber Cooking

BEANS ARE THE FIBER CHAMPIONS

Beans are loaded with fiber. If you are using canned beans, you can reduce their sodium content by choosing reduced-sodium brands or draining the liquid and rinsing the beans before serving them. If you use dried beans, cooking is usually more time-consuming, but you'll avoid added sodium, and they are considerably less expensive and more flavorful than the canned varieties. See table 3 for cooking instructions and the yield of dried beans.

TABLE 3 Cooking yield of dried beans

LEGUME (1 cup dried)	WATER:BEAN RATIO	COOKING TIME	YIELD (after soaking and cooking)
adzuki (aduki) beans	4:1	45 min.	3 cups
black (turtle) beans	3:1	1–1½ hr.	3 cups
black-eyed peas	3:1	30 min.	2½ cups
chickpeas (garbanzo beans)	4:1	1–1½ hr.	3 cups
great northern beans	3:1	1–1½ hr.	2⅔ cups
kidney or red beans	3:1	1–1½ hr.	2¾ cups
lentils, brown	2:1	30 min.	3 cups
lentils, green	2:1	30–45 min.	2 cups
lentils, red	2:1	15–20 min.	3 cups
lima beans	3:1	1 hr.	3 cups
mung beans	3:1	45 min.	3 cups
navy (pea) or small white beans	3:1	45–60 min.	2¾ cups
pinto or pink beans	3:1	45–60 min.	3¼ cups
soybeans	4:1	2–3 hr.	2¾ cups
split peas, green or yellow	4:1	45–60 min.	2 cups

Replacing Home-Cooked Beans with Canned Beans

Using canned beans can save time and energy when you are on a tight schedule. To replace 1½ cups of home-cooked beans in any recipe, use 1 can (15 ounces) of canned beans. To reduce the sodium content of canned beans that contain salt, drain the beans in a colander, rinse them well, and drain again before using.

Taming the Wild Bean: Easing Digestion

If beans give you a bit of indigestion or gas, here are some tips that will solve this problem:

1. Start with modest servings. Also, some people notice that smaller beans are easier to digest, so try black beans, black-eyed peas, and lentils first, and then work your way up to pinto and fava beans.
2. Make sure the beans are thoroughly cooked. Adding a strip of kombu, a sea vegetable, to the beans during cooking can also be helpful.
3. Drain and gently rinse canned beans. This also decreases the amount of salt in some brands.
4. Before cooking, soak dried beans for 8 to 12 hours in cold water, or 2 to 4 hours in warm water (bring to a boil, remove from the heat, cover, and let rest at room temperature). After soaking dried beans, drain and cook them in enough fresh water to keep them covered by several inches. Beans can take a very long time to cook (up to several hours), and the length of time necessary to reach tenderness depends on several factors: (1) water hardness, (2) size of the bean, (3) age of the bean, (4) and cooking method (for example, pressure cooking cuts the time significantly, by about two-thirds or more).

Recommended Recipes

Calabacitas (p. 175)
Low-Fat Guacamole (p. 110)
Mango Salsa (p. 111)
Quick Bean Burritos (p. 207)

To Do This Week

Drop by any large grocery store and take a look at the beans they carry. You'll notice they are found in three different aisles: First, you'll find bags of dried beans in a surprising range of varieties. Then, in the canned vegetables section, you'll find baked beans, limas, and other types. And in the "ethnic" or "international" aisle, you'll find Italian varieties (such as chickpeas and cannellini beans), Mexican refried beans, and perhaps other types. Select at least one new bean variety or product and give it a try this week. If you're not too big on beans, start with small servings to avoid gassiness.

TABLE 4 Grains cooking chart

GRAIN (1 cup dry)	GRAIN:WATER RATIO	COOKING TIME	YIELD (after soaking and cooking)
amaranth	1:2½	20–25 min.	2½ cups
barley, flakes	1:2	30–40 min.	2½ cups
barley, hulled	1:3	1¼ hr.	3½ cups
barley, pearl	1:3	50–60 min.	3½ cups
buckwheat groats	1:2	15 min.	2½ cups
cornmeal (fine)	1:4–4½	8–10 min.	2½ cups
cornmeal (polenta, coarse)	1:4–4½	20–25 min.	2½ cups
millet, hulled	1:3–4	20–25 min.	3½ cups
oat, bran or quick oats	1:2½	5 min.	2 cups
oat, groats/whole	1:3	30–40 min.	3½ cups
oats, rolled	1:1¾	15 min.	3 cups
oats, steel-cut, Scotch or Irish	1:2½	30–45 min.	3 cups
quinoa	1:2	15–20 min.	2¾ cups
rice, brown basmati	1:2½	35–40 min.	3 cups
rice, brown, long-grain	1:2½	45–55 min.	3 cups
rice, brown, short-grain	1:2	45–55 min.	3 cups
rice, wild	1:3	50–60 min.	4 cups
rye, berries	1:3½	60 min.	3 cups
rye, flakes	1:2	10–15 min.	3 cups
spelt	1:3½	40–50 min.	2½ cups
teff	1:3	5–20 min.	3½ cups
triticale	1:3	1¾ hr.	2½ cups
wheat, bulgur	1:2	15 min.	2½ cups
wheat, couscous	1:1	5 min.	2 cups
wheat, cracked	1:2	20–25 min.	2½ cups
wheat, whole berries	1:3	2 hr.	2½ cups

While you're there, pick up a package of whole-grain rice—that is, brown rice. Brown rice retains the natural grain fiber missing from white rice. Grains make a wonderful accompaniment to beans. Their wide variety and diverse flavors, and the fact that they are so inexpensive, make grains an exciting new food group to explore. Experiment with the different types found in your grocery store, and use the amounts and times in table 4 to guide you in your preparations.

Discovering
Dairy Alternatives

Most North Americans and Europeans grow up with the idea that milk is a healthful beverage, and the dairy industry has certainly done its best to promote that idea. However, researchers seeking to understand why people following Western diets tend to have high cancer rates have begun to blame not only meat and other fatty foods, but also dairy products.

In 1998, Harvard researchers reported findings in a large group of health professionals. Those who typically consumed more than two servings of milk per day had a 60 percent increased risk of prostate cancer compared to those who generally avoided milk.[1] Two years later, a Harvard study on another large group of men showed much the same thing—milk drinkers had significantly more prostate cancer.[2] Many other studies have had similar findings, and researchers have also examined the role of dairy products—positive or negative—in other forms of cancer.

Why would dairy products influence cancer risk? Is the problem due to hormones or other chemicals in milk, or is it due to the basic nutrient makeup of milk—its fat or protein, perhaps? What does this mean for people who have been diagnosed with cancer already? And if milk does have health risks, what should we use instead?

Milk and Cancer Risk

To understand why dairy products might play a role in cancer, it helps to remember their biological purpose. Milk is produced by mothers to support the rapid growth of their newborns. It contains plenty of protein, fat, and sugar (lactose), as well as dozens of hormones and other natural chemical substances that direct infants' growth and development. Milk differs from species to species—cow's milk is quite different in its nutrient profile from human milk—but all mammals' milk is designed to encourage rapid growth.

People following Western diets tend to have high cancer rates and have begun to blame not only meat and other fatty foods, but also dairy products.

17

After the age of weaning, of course, all mammals stop drinking their mothers' milk. A few thousand years ago, however, humans began to domesticate animals and to consume milk taken from cows and a few other mammals.

When humans drink cow's milk, it causes some worrisome biological changes in the body, one of which is a rise in the amount of insulin-like growth factor 1 (IGF-1) in the bloodstream.[3,4] IGF-1 is a powerful stimulus for cancer cell growth. When breast cancer cells are mixed with IGF-1 in a test tube, for example, they grow rapidly.

Milk drinkers have more IGF-1 in their bloodstreams. IGF-1 is a powerful stimulus for cancer cell growth.

Researchers have known for many years that men and women with higher levels of IGF-1 in their blood are at higher risk for prostate and premenopausal breast cancer, respectively, compared to those with lower levels.[5,6] So one way that milk may influence cancer risk is by increasing the amount of IGF-1 in the blood. Individuals who have been diagnosed with cancer may be quite right to be concerned that milk drinking boosts IGF-1 levels in their bloodstreams, given that IGF-1, in turn, can encourage cancer cell growth.

Milk causes other chemical changes in the body as well, some of which relate to specific types of cancer. Generally speaking, these mechanisms relate not only to the likelihood that cancer will strike, but also to how rapidly it will grow and spread once it has occurred.

Prostate Cancer

Large studies have shown that milk-drinking men have a higher risk of prostate cancer. However, milk's ability to boost IGF-1 is not the only mechanism by which this occurs. Milk is also high in fat and has no fiber at all. As a result, it may increase the body's production of testosterone, which is linked to prostate cancer risk.

In addition, milk appears to interfere with the activation of vitamin D in the body. Vitamin D is actually a hormone that helps your body absorb calcium from the digestive tract. It also protects the prostate against cancer. Vitamin D is normally produced by sunlight's action on the skin. Although it can also come from the diet, edible forms of the vitamin are inactive precursors. In order to function as full-fledged vitamin D, the substance must pass first to the liver and then to the kidneys for slight changes to its molecular structure. This is where dairy products become a problem. As the load of calcium from ingested dairy products floods into the bloodstream, it apparently signals the body that, since there is plenty of calcium in the system already, the body does not need to activate vitamin D to try to absorb any more. That is, the body reduces its vitamin D activation so that it does not absorb *too much* calcium, since calcium overdoses can be toxic.

The result: High-calcium foods can cause a substantial drop in the amount of activated vitamin D in the blood. And since vitamin D is essential for maintaining a healthy prostate, less vitamin D in the blood may mean that the risk of prostate cancer climbs. Researchers have found that less vitamin D in the blood is indeed associated with higher cancer risk. Milk often contains added vitamin D, but it is in the inactive precursor form, and dairy consumption suppresses vitamin D activation in the body.[1]

At least twenty research reports in diverse populations, including the Harvard studies mentioned above, have linked milk drinking to prostate cancer. In addition, two recent meta-analyses that evaluated the combined results of twelve prospective studies and eleven case-control studies found a consistent positive association with both dairy intake and calcium intake on prostate cancer risk.[7,8]

Other Cancers

Researchers at Harvard University and elsewhere have also studied the links between milk consumption and ovarian cancer, but with mixed results. The hypotheses under scrutiny have related not only to milk's fat content, but also to its sugar, *lactose*.

Lactose is actually made of two smaller sugar molecules called *galactose* and *glucose*. When these two sugars are split apart—either by the bacteria used to produce yogurt or by digestive enzymes in your intestinal tract—galactose and glucose enter the blood. Galactose may be the problem. In large concentrations, galactose may be toxic to the ovaries, encouraging infertility and possibly cancer. A recent analysis of studies examining a relationship between dairy product consumption (skim, low-fat, and whole milk, yogurt, cheese, and lactose) and ovarian cancer risk found that for every 10 grams of lactose consumed (the amount in one glass of milk), ovarian cancer risk increased by 13 percent among the prospective cohort studies.[9]

Women with higher levels of IGF-1 in their blood have a greater risk of premenopausal breast cancer. The Harvard Nurses' Health Study found that women with higher IGF-1 levels had more than double the risk compared to women with lower IGF-1 levels.[6] Other researchers have made similar findings.[10] As we've seen, milk drinking raises IGF-1 levels.

Other studies seeking to nail down the links between dairy consumption and breast cancer risk have yielded mixed results, with some finding higher risk of breast cancer among milk drinkers and others finding no such association.

Foods that are high in calcium appear to reduce colon cancer risk. However, people seeking ways to use calcium-rich foods to reduce colon cancer risk would do well to get their calcium from green leafy vegetables and beans rather than from dairy products. Prostate and breast cancer are more common than colon cancer. Using dairy products to try to reduce colon cancer risk may increase the risk of other, more common cancers.

More Healthful Beverages

There is no shortage of better beverages. Soymilk, rice milk, almond milk, and oat milk come in a wide variety of flavors and work very well on cereal or for drinking. They are available in calcium-enriched and regular versions, and many have additional vitamin fortification. Because a number of these products require no refrigeration until they are opened (if they are packaged in aseptic cartons), grocery stores sometimes stock them on the dry goods shelves rather than in the refrigerated section.

The Most Healthful Calcium Sources

Green leafy vegetables and legumes (beans, peas, and lentils) contain calcium and, unlike milk, are rich in fiber and other nutrients that protect against cancer. You'll also find plenty of calcium in supplements and, as we've mentioned, in fortified soymilk and similar products. Calcium-fortified juices are now widely available. However, it is important to remember that increased calcium intake may be one of the reasons why milk is linked to prostate cancer (because high calcium intakes interfere with vitamin D activation). If that is true, you should be equally cautious about *any* product that is extremely high in calcium, including fortified foods and supplements. In that light, green leafy vegetables and beans are your best calcium sources. They have adequate calcium, but not excessive amounts.

However, don't depend on calcium alone—from any source—to protect you from osteoporosis. While the dairy industry has pushed drinking milk as a means of preventing the bone-thinning condition, studies show that the strategy is largely useless.

Researchers at Pennsylvania State University found that for girls in their peak bone-building years—ages twelve to eighteen—getting extra calcium made no difference at all in bone growth.[11] Exercise worked very well to foster bone growth, but extra calcium did not. Similarly, in a Harvard study, a group of 72,337 postmenopausal women followed for eighteen years showed that dairy calcium did not help bone strength at all. Women who got the most calcium from dairy sources actually had no protection against hip fracture compared to those who got little or no dairy calcium.[12]

So how do you protect your bones? Here are the most important factors to remember:

- Exercise is the first key. Your bones need a reason to live, so to speak—and exercise strengthens them noticeably.
- Vitamin D—from sunlight or vitamin supplements—helps keep bones strong.

- While you do need calcium, studies have not shown substantial benefits of intakes higher than about 600 milligrams per day for healthy adults.
- Fruits and vegetables provide vitamin C to build collagen, which forms the basic network of tissue within your bones.

TABLE 5 Calcium in plant foods

FOOD	SERVING SIZE	CALCIUM CONTENT	FRACTIONAL ABSORPTION	ESTIMATED ABSORBABLE CALCIUM PER SERVING
almonds, dry roasted	1 ounce	80 mg	21%	17 mg
beans, great northern or navy	1 cup	121–128 mg	17%	21–22 mg
beans, pinto or red	1 cup	82-89 mg	17%	14–15 mg
beans, white	1 cup	161 mg	17%	27 mg
broccoli, boiled	1 cup	178 mg	53%	94 mg
brussels sprouts, boiled	1 cup	56 mg	64%	36 mg
cabbage, green, boiled	1 cup	50 mg	65%	33 mg
cauliflower, boiled	1 cup	34 mg	69%	23 mg
Chinese cabbage, boiled	1 cup	158 mg	54%	85 mg
collard greens, boiled	1 cup	358 mg	52%	186 mg
figs, dried	10 medium	135 mg	n/a	n/a
kale, boiled	1 cup	188 mg	59%	111 mg
mustard greens, boiled	1 cup	152 mg	58%	88 mg
orange juice, calcium-fortified	1 cup	300 mg	38%	114 mg
rice milk, calcium-fortified	1 cup	300 mg	24%	72 mg
rutabaga, boiled	1 cup	72 mg	61%	44 mg
sesame seed butter (tahini)	1 tablespoon	64 mg	21%	13 mg
sesame seeds, unhulled	1 ounce	381 mg	21%	58 mg
soymilk, calcium-fortified	1 cup	300 mg	24%	72 mg
spinach, boiled*	1 cup	244 mg	5%	12 mg
tofu, set with calcium, firm	½ cup	258 mg	31%	80 mg
turnip greens, boiled	1 cup	198 mg	52%	103 mg

* Spinach contains oxalic acid, which hinders calcium absorption. Other dark leafy greens, such as kale, mustard greens, bok choy, and cabbage, are better sources of calcium.

Sources: Weaver C. M., W. R. Proulx, and R. Heaney. Choices for achieving adequate dietary calcium with a vegetarian diet. *Am J Clin Nutr.* 1999; 70(suppl):543S–548S. • Weaver C. M., and K. L. Plawecki. Dietary calcium: adequacy of a vegetarian diet. *Am J Clin Nutr.* 1994;59(suppl): 1238S–1241S. • Keller J. L., A. J. Lanou, and N. D. Barnard. The consumer cost of calcium from food and supplements. *J Am Diet Assoc.* 2002;102:1669–1671.

Perhaps most important of all, you should understand that osteoporosis is usually not a condition of inadequate calcium intake. Rather, *it is a condition of overly rapid calcium loss*. Three factors, in particular, accelerate calcium losses, and controlling them gives you important power against osteoporosis:

- Sodium (salt) accelerates the passage of calcium through the kidneys into the urine. To reduce sodium intake, be careful about consuming processed or canned foods and snack products made with added sodium.
- Animal protein is high in *sulfur-containing amino acids*, which tend to leach calcium from the bones and send it through the kidneys into the urine.
- Smokers have rapid calcium losses.

Meal Planning

- Include calcium-rich greens (such as kale, collard greens, mustard greens, turnip greens, bok choy, and broccoli) and beans in your routine. Add greens and/or beans to stir-fries, sauces, salads, and casseroles.
- Have calcium-rich snacks, such as figs, raisins, almonds, and dates.
- Replace cow's milk with nondairy alternatives, such as soymilk, rice milk, almond milk, or oat milk, in meals and recipes.
- Sprinkle nutritional yeast on pasta and other main dishes for a healthful, cheesy-tasting alternative to dairy cheese.
- Try fresh fruit sorbets and nondairy frozen desserts instead of ice cream or frozen yogurt.
- Enjoy oatmeal and other calcium-rich breakfast cereals with fresh fruit and nondairy milk alternatives for breakfast.

Recommended Recipes

Chocolate Mousse (page 215)
Cream of Broccoli Soup (page 122)
Penne with Kale, Tomatoes, and Olives (page 196)
White Bean Spread with Sun-Dried Tomatoes (page 119)

To Do This Week

Did you ever switch from whole milk to skim or nonfat milk? How did the new version taste at first? For many people, fat-reduced milks taste watery and a bit "off" at first. But after two or three weeks, what happened? The new milk tasted perfectly fine, didn't it? And if you ever went back to whole milk, what was it like then? Chances are, it seemed too thick and fatty—almost like paint.

It takes only a couple of weeks for your taste buds to accommodate to new tastes. So if you try rice milk or another nondairy beverage, it will probably not taste quite right at first. But within a week or two, it will taste perfectly fine.

This week, take a trip to the natural food store (or a large, well-stocked grocery store). If you normally drink cow's milk or add it to cereal, pick up a few different brands of rice or almond milk and give them a try. Notice that they come in regular, vanilla, chocolate, and perhaps other flavors, as well as low-fat varieties enriched with vitamins and calcium.

If you are a fan of yogurt, ice cream, sour cream, or cheese, natural food stores stock nondairy alternatives for them, too. Some are more flavorful than others, so try a few different types and brands and see which ones appeal to you.

Replacing Meat

When cancer researchers started to look for links between diet and cancer, one of the most noticeable findings was that people who avoided meat were less likely to develop the disease. Large studies in England and Germany showed that vegetarians were about 40 percent less likely to develop cancer compared to meat eaters.[1,2,3] In the United States, researchers studied Seventh-day Adventists. This religious group is remarkable because, although nearly all members avoid tobacco and alcohol and follow generally healthful lifestyles, about half of the Adventist population is vegetarian, while the others consume fairly modest amounts of meat. This fact allowed scientists to separate the effects of eating meat from other factors. Overall, these studies showed significant reductions in cancer risk among those who avoided meat.[4]

Time and again, research points to red and processed meat consumption as significantly increasing colorectal cancer risk when compared to the diets of people who generally avoid these foods.[5,6] In the Cancer Prevention Study II, which involved 148,610 adults followed since 1982, the group with the highest red meat intake had approximately 30–40 percent higher colon cancer risk, and the group with the highest processed meat intake had approximately 50 percent higher colon cancer risk compared to those with lower intakes.[7] In this study, high red meat intake was defined as three ounces of beef, lamb, or pork for men and two ounces for women daily. For comparison, a typical hamburger contains four ounces of beef. Earlier studies have also indicated that those who consume white meat, particularly chicken, have approximately a threefold higher colon cancer risk compared to vegetarians,[8] although other studies have not confirmed this finding.

There is limited research evaluating the role of diet and colon cancer survival; however, in a new study of 1,009 colon cancer patients, researchers found that survival depended to a great extent on dietary habits. Those who consumed more red and processed meats, sweets, and refined grains were

Large research studies have shown that vegetarians are about 40 percent less likely to develop cancer compared to meat eaters.

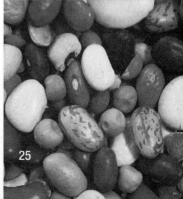

more likely to have a recurrence of or die from the disease after a median five-year follow-up, while those who consumed more fruits, vegetables, whole grains, and less red and processed meats and refined foods were less likely to experience a recurrence and more likely to survive.[9]

Why Is Meat Linked to Cancer?

Why should meat contribute to cancer risk? For starters, its fat content is virtually always much higher than that of plant products. Even skinless chicken breast harbors a surprising amount of fat, and virtually all meats are totally out of the league of truly low-fat foods—whole grains, beans, vegetables, and fruits.

Since meat is not a plant product, it never has any fiber at all. The more you fill up on meat, the less room you have for fiber-rich foods. As we discovered in chapter 1, fatty, low-fiber foods boost the hormones that are linked to common forms of cancer. Meat is also devoid of vitamin C and low in other protective nutrients found in plants.

Researchers have started to investigate additional reasons that link meat to cancer risk. Scientists in London found that individuals who consumed a diet high in red meat (15 ounces per day) had significantly higher colon levels of N-nitroso compounds—compounds that can alter DNA and increase the risk of developing colon cancer—compared to the levels found in those who consumed a vegetarian diet. An intermediate group that consumed red meat and high-fiber foods had lower levels of N-nitroso compounds than those eating the high-meat diet, but not as low as the vegetarian group. This suggests that fiber may have played a protective role for the intermediate group by repairing damaged DNA and decreasing the amount of time harmful compounds, such as N-nitroso compounds, stay in the colon.[10]

Meat also has other problems. As meats are cooked, cancer-causing chemicals called heterocyclic amines tend to form within the meat tissue, as we saw in chapter 2. The longer and hotter meat is cooked, the more these compounds form. Grilled chicken has turned out to harbor these cancer-causing substances and is the largest source of heterocyclic amines in the U.S. diet.[11]

More Healthful Protein Sources

Some people think of meat as their main source of protein. But it is easy to get plenty of protein without the fat, cholesterol, and other undesirables in meat.

Beans, vegetables, and whole grains, in particular, have more than enough protein to sustain a health-promoting diet. The American Dietetic Association's guidelines state that a diet including a variety of these healthful plant foods provides all the protein you need.[12] In years past, some people thought that vegetarians had to eat foods in certain combinations—grains with beans, for example—in order to get adequate protein. However, it turns out that no special combining is necessary. A diet including a variety of beans, vegetables, and whole grains will easily give you more than enough protein, even without intentional combining of foods.

Meal Planning

So, how do we replace meat? In many recipes, the legume group comes to your rescue. Beans and lentils, for example, add heartiness to soups, stews, chili, and other recipes. When making burritos, leave out the ground beef and use vegetarian refried beans. Despite their name, low-fat "refried" beans are not really fried; they are actually just mashed pinto beans. You'll find them in the Mexican food section of your local grocery store. They are satisfying and loaded with fiber and protein; you'll never miss the meat.

The American Dietetic Association's guidelines state that a diet including a variety of healthful plant foods provides all the protein you need.

Portobello mushrooms also make great meat alternatives. They have a meaty texture and savory flavor, especially after being marinated in low-fat dressing and then grilled or heated in a frying pan. Use portobello mushrooms as "burgers" at your next barbecue or to fill the meat layer in your lasagne.

Seitan is a fascinating product derived from wheat protein. It has been used to simulate virtually every kind of cold cut or meaty dish imaginable. It has a hearty texture and makes a nutritious meat substitute. Wheat protein is also the main ingredient in a number of meat analogs, including spicy veggie pepperoni and sausages.

Soy products have been turned into endless varieties of hot dogs, burgers, and other simulated meats. Many of these products taste so much like the real thing that they will help you break a meat habit. Properly chosen, they will also greatly reduce the fat content of your diet. Some researchers have suggested that soy has special cancer-fighting properties, although investigations in this area are not yet sufficient to support this possibility. For now, soy's proven virtue is its ability to pry people away from meat.

Note: If you are taking any breast cancer medications, please consult your doctor before consuming any processed soy foods, even if they are meat substitutions. (For more on this topic, see page 80, under "Soy.")

Recommended Recipes

Ambrosia (page 213)
Chickpea Burgers (page 204)
Easy Bean Salad (page 140)
Tempeh Broccoli Sauté (page 201)

To Do This Week

1. Check out meat substitutes at a natural food store and try one or more of them. Try a sampling of veggie burgers, hot dogs, and deli slices or, if you prefer, the many varieties of beans and lentils.
2. Turn three of your favorite recipes into meatless meals using beans, seitan, mushrooms, tofu, tempeh, or other meat substitutes.

Cancer-Fighting Compounds and Immune-Boosting Foods

As you push your grocery cart down the aisle, you'll want to keep a lookout for foods that have special cancer-fighting properties. In this chapter, we'll focus on foods rich in protective compounds called *antioxidants* and *phytochemicals*, as well as foods that can help boost your immune system.

As you plan your menu, you'll want to be generous with a variety of vegetables and fruits, because they are the main sources of these healthful compounds. Studies have amply demonstrated the ability of diets rich in vegetables and fruits to reduce the likelihood that cancer will develop in the first place. Although fewer studies have investigated their effect on survival after diagnosis, some have suggested that cancer survivors who consume more vegetables and fruits do indeed live longer. As you'll see, researchers have begun to tease out reasons why produce is so powerful.[1,2]

Antioxidants

To understand antioxidants, let's start with how oxygen works in the body. Every minute of every day, we breathe in oxygen and breathe out carbon dioxide. Although oxygen is used for a variety of vitally important functions in the body, it happens to be a very unstable molecule. In the course of the normal chemical reactions that occur in the bloodstream or inside our cells, oxygen can easily be damaged, which is to say it can lose some of its electrons or perhaps gain some. While electrons normally orbit a molecule's nucleus in as calm and orderly a fashion as the moon circles Earth, oxygen's electrons can slip into off-kilter orbits.

The point is that we have millions of oxygen molecules in our bodies, and they easily become unstable. When that happens, they become like piranhas, ready to take a bite out of the cells that make up your skin, blood vessels, internal organs, or any other part of your body. These piranhas—these unstable and dangerous oxygen molecules—are called *free radicals*.

As you plan your menu, be generous with a variety of vegetables and fruits, because they are the main sources of these healthful compounds.

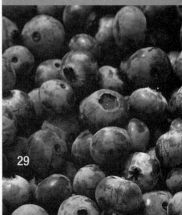

29

They can even attack your *chromosomes*, the strands of DNA that lie deep within your cells and hold all the genes that make you who you are. When oxygen free radicals damage chromosomes, cells can lose their ability to control their basic functions. They can begin to multiply out of control, and that is the beginning of cancer. Biologists believe that much of the aging process and many cancers are caused by free radical damage.

Plants can be damaged by oxygen free radicals too, so nature has given them the ability to produce natural compounds that act like shields to defend against these wild oxygen molecules. You can see why these natural compounds are called antioxidants—they protect the plant from oxygen free radicals. And when you eat plants, their antioxidants enter your bloodstream and act to protect you, too. When all goes well, the free radicals—the unstable oxygen molecules—attack the antioxidants and leave your cells and chromosomes alone in the same way that a bullet might dent the hardened surface of an armored car but spare the occupants inside.

Beta-Carotene

One of the best-known antioxidants is *beta-carotene*, the yellow-orange pigment found in carrots, yams, and cantaloupes. Beta-carotene has long been looked on kindly by nutritionists because it provides vitamin A, which is important for good vision, among other functions. Beta-carotene is actually two molecules of vitamin A joined together.

However, beta-carotene does more than simply provide vitamin A. It enters the cell membrane that surrounds each of the cells that make up your body and then waits there to fend off free radicals that might approach.

Beta-carotene also has a measurable immune-boosting effect with as little as 30 milligrams of beta-carotene per day—the amount in two large carrots.[3,4] Dietary reference intakes are set for vitamin A, rather than its precursor, beta-carotene. However, the Institute of Medicine holds that 3–6 milligrams of beta-carotene per day—equivalent to 800–1,700 IU (240–510 retinol equivalents) of vitamin A—is sufficient to maintain beta-carotene blood levels in the range associated with a lower risk of chronic diseases.[5]

Beta-carotene enters the cell membrane that surrounds each of your cells and protects the cell from free radical damage.

You'll find beta-carotene not only in orange-colored fruits and vegetables; it is also in dark green leafy vegetables. You can't see the orange color because the green chlorophyll hides beta-carotene in the same way that chlorophyll in tree leaves hides the plants' underlying orange, red, and brown colors until the green color fades in autumn. For a list of foods rich in beta-carotene, check table 6 (page 31).

Although you can buy beta-carotene supplements, it is much better to get beta-carotene from foods. In fact, studies testing beta-carotene's cancer-

TABLE 6 Beta-carotene in selected foods

FOOD	SERVING SIZE	AMOUNT OF BETA-CAROTENE
cantaloupe	1 cup	3 mg
carrot	1 large	16 mg
kale	1 cup	4 mg
mango	1 cup	4 mg
pumpkin	1 cup	32 mg
yam	1 cup	26 mg

Source: U.S. Department of Agriculture, Agricultural Research Service. 2007. USDA National Nutrient Database for Standard Reference, Release 20. Nutrient Data Laboratory Home Page, *www.nal.usda.gov/fnic/foodcomp.*

fighting power in smokers (a group selected because they are at particular risk for cancer) showed that those whose diets were high in beta-carotene had a measure of protection, but those who got beta-carotene from supplements were actually *more likely to develop cancer* than were other smokers. The reason is not entirely clear, but it may be that, since supplements deliver high doses of only one antioxidant, they interfere with the absorption of others. Moreover, vegetables and fruits that are rich in beta-carotene are loaded with hundreds of additional antioxidants, vitamins, minerals, and other protective compounds.

The moral of the story is that there is plenty of beta-carotene in vegetables and fruits, and they are the best sources.

Lycopene

You may not have heard much about *lycopene*, but you have certainly seen plenty of it. Just as beta-carotene is nature's yellow-orange pigment, lycopene is a bright red pigment, providing the color for tomatoes, watermelon, and pink grapefruit.

Lycopene is in the *carotenoid* family, meaning that it is beta-carotene's chemical cousin, and it is actually a much more powerful antioxidant. A study at Harvard University showed that men who had just two servings of tomato sauce per week had 23 percent less prostate cancer risk compared to those who rarely had tomato products.[6] Men consuming ten or more servings of tomato products each week had a 35 percent reduction in risk, and that was true *even if their tomatoes came in the form of pizza sauce, spaghetti sauce, or ketchup.* In fact, the cooking process releases lycopene from the plant's cells, increasing our ability to absorb it.

Men who had ten or more servings of tomato products each week had a 35 percent reduction in prostate cancer risk.

TABLE 7 Lycopene in selected foods

FOOD	SERVING SIZE	AMOUNT OF LYCOPENE
pink grapefruit	1 medium	5 mg
tomato, raw	1 medium	4 mg
tomato juice	1 cup	23 mg
tomato ketchup	1 tablespoon	3 mg
tomato-based spaghetti sauce	½ cup	20 mg
watermelon	1 slice (280 g)	14 mg

Source: Heinz Institute of Nutritional Sciences, *www.lycopene.org.*

Not all red foods contain lycopene, however, as nature has a couple of other similar pigments in its paint box. The red color in strawberries, for example, does not come from lycopene, but from a group of pigments called *anthocyanins*, which are powerful antioxidants in their own right. (Other anthocyanins provide the color for blueberries, cherries, plums, and red cabbage.) Table 7 lists the top foods for lycopene.

Vitamin E and Selenium

Vitamin E and the mineral selenium are also part of your antioxidant arsenal. Like beta-carotene and lycopene, they protect each cell's outer membrane from free radical attacks. Vitamin E is found in legumes (beans), whole grains, and plants rich in natural oils (such as nuts and seeds).

However, while a little bit of vitamin E is good—in fact, it is an essential part of your body's protection against free radicals—it is not at all certain that boosting vitamin E intake to high levels is a good idea. Some of the richest vitamin E sources, such as vegetable oils and nuts, also give you an unwanted load of fat. This may be the reason why one study found that, among women with breast cancer, those with the highest levels of vitamin E in their bloodstreams were actually *more likely* to succumb to the disease than those with more moderate levels; this may simply be a sign that they were getting too much fat in their diets.[7] So while more research is needed to sort out what is the right amount of vitamin E, it is prudent to choose foods that are moderate in the vitamin, rather than extremely high or low. These foods are listed in table 8.

In addition, researchers have found that individuals eating vitamin E–rich foods also tend to have improved immunity. But increasing vitamin E intake to high levels through supplements can impair immune function.[8] The best advice appears to be to stick with food sources and avoid vitamin E supplements.

The amount of selenium in plants varies depending on the amount present in the soil where they grow. But, given modern food distribution

TABLE 8 Good sources of vitamin E and selenium

FOOD	AMOUNT	VITAMIN E	SELENIUM
barley, cooked	1 cup	3 mg	36 mcg
Brazil nuts	3 nuts	1 mg	420 mcg
broccoli, raw	1 cup	2 mg	3 mcg
brown rice, cooked	1 cup	1 mg	14 mcg
brussels sprouts, cooked	1 cup	1 mg	2 mcg
chickpeas, cooked	1 cup	2 mg	6 mcg
garlic, raw	3 cloves	.01 mg	1.3 mcg
pinto beans, cooked	1 cup	2 mg	12 mcg
pumpkin, cooked	1 cup	3 mg	1 mcg
sunflower seeds, raw	1 tablespoon	5 mg	5 mcg

Source: U.S. Department of Agriculture, Agricultural Research Service. 2007. USDA National Nutrient Database for Standard Reference, Release 20. Nutrient Data Laboratory Home Page, *www.nal.usda.gov/fnic/foodcomp.*

patterns, your rice is likely to come from one place, your beans from another, and so on. So your selenium intake is likely to be reasonably generous if you include grains and legumes in your daily routine.

Vitamin C

Vitamin C is a powerful and well-known antioxidant. But unlike the other antioxidants we've looked at so far, which defend cell membranes, vitamin C patrols the watery areas of the body—the bloodstream or the cell's interior.

Nobel laureate Linus Pauling was a strong advocate for vitamin C, and research suggests that, indeed, vitamin C boosts immunity, in addition to its antioxidant abilities. Once again, vegetables and fruits are the preferred sources. The recommended daily intake is only 90 milligrams per day for men and 75 milligrams per day for women. However, some researchers have recommended higher amounts, typically in the form of supplements and usually in the neighborhood of 500–2,000 milligrams. There appear to be no adverse effects from these higher doses of vitamin C.

What are the best foods for vitamin C? Well, citrus fruits are famous for it, but you'll find surprisingly large amounts in many vegetables. Table 9 lists some good sources.

Phytochemicals

While antioxidants have the job of protecting you from the free radicals, plants have many other protective substances, too. Biologists call them

TABLE 9 Good sources of vitamin C

FOOD	AMOUNT	VITAMIN C
bell pepper, red, raw	1 cup	175 mg
broccoli, raw	1 cup	82 mg
brussels sprouts, cooked	1 cup	97 mg
cantaloupe	1 cup	68 mg
guava	1 cup	303 mg
kiwi	1 cup	164 mg
lemon	1 medium	83 mg
orange	1 medium	59 mg
orange juice	½ cup	124 mg
strawberries	1 cup	82 mg

Source: U.S. Department of Agriculture, Agricultural Research Service. 2007. USDA National Nutrient Database for Standard Reference, Release 20. Nutrient Data Laboratory Home Page, *http://www.nal.usda.gov/fnic/foodcomp.*

phytochemicals. "Phyto" comes from the Greek word *phyton,* which means "plant," so phytochemicals are simply natural chemicals found in plants.

Although researchers first turned their attention to these chemicals because of their apparent ability to prevent cancer, the possibility that these natural compounds can also enhance survival after cancer has been diagnosed is also now under study. Two groups are especially good to get to know: *cruciferous* vegetables and the *allium* family of vegetables.

Cruciferous vegetables, such as broccoli, cabbage, and collard greens, get their name from the cross-shaped flowers that adorn them just before the plants go to seed. People who eat generous amounts of these vegetables have remarkably low cancer rates, and researchers have dedicated a great deal of effort to isolating the compounds that are responsible for their anticancer effects.

Broccoli, for example, contains *sulforaphane,* a compound that augments the liver's ability to rid the body of toxic chemicals and excrete carcinogenic compounds.[9] Other phytochemicals in broccoli and other cruciferous vegetables have demonstrated the ability to arrest the growth of cancer cells.[2,10]

Cruciferous vegetables also affect the hormones that influence the progression of hormone-dependent cancers, such as breast cancer. In particular, these vegetables actually change the way estrogens are broken down and eliminated.

Cruciferous Vegetables

arugula	kale
bok choy	kohlrabi
broccoli	mustard greens
brussels sprouts	radishes
cabbage	rutabaga
cauliflower	turnip greens
collard greens	turnips
horseradish	watercress

Normally, estradiol—a potent estrogen in a woman's bloodstream—is converted to *16 α-hydroxyestrone*, a hormone that encourages the growth of cancer cells. However, the cruciferous extract *indole-3-carbinol* causes the body to convert more estrogen to a different estrogen called *2-hydroxyestrone*, which has anticancer actions.[11]

Researchers are starting to test out the effects of cruciferous vegetable extracts on patients. In one study, the extract indole-3-carbinol was given to women with abnormal cervical cells (the type of cells gynecologists check for on Pap smears). After twelve weeks, the abnormal cells had disappeared in half the treated patients, while patients given a placebo preparation showed no improvement.[11]

Because some vegetables, such as broccoli, are difficult to digest in their raw state, you may be wondering if cooking knocks out their protective effects. Studies show that, while cooking does indeed reduce the amount of phytochemicals in vegetables, it does not eliminate them.[2]

The *allium* group of vegetables includes garlic, onions, and hundreds of their botanical relatives. Yes, chefs value their flavors, but researchers are increasingly intrigued by the possibility that they may speed the body's elimination of carcinogens and perhaps even block the start of cancer or inhibit the growth of cancer cells.

Allium Vegetables		
chives	green onions	onions
garlic	leeks	shallots

Garlic, in particular, has been subjected to a great deal of scientific study. When garlic cloves are cut or crushed, they produce a compound called *allicin*, which is responsible for both their scent and their biological activity. Several studies have shown that people who regularly include allium vegetables in their diets have less risk of cancer, particularly cancers of the stomach and colon.[12] In test-tube experiments, extracts from these plants have been shown to help eliminate carcinogens and slow the growth of cancer cells.[13] Researchers estimate the amount of garlic necessary for anticancer effects is three to five cloves daily.[14] Cooking temperatures eliminate garlic's beneficial effects on cells unless the garlic is allowed to stand for about ten minutes between being crushed and the cooking process.[15]

TABLE 10 Antioxidant minimum daily target

ANTIOXIDANT	WOMEN (14–70< Y)	MEN (14–70< Y)
beta-carotene	800 mcg	1,000 mcg
selenium	55 mcg	55 mcg
vitamin C	75 mg	90 mg
vitamin E	15 mg	15 mg

TABLE 11 Antioxidants in vegetables

VEGETABLE	SERVING SIZE	BETA-CAROTENE	SELENIUM	VITAMIN C	VITAMIN E
broccoli, raw	1 cup	807 mcg	3 mcg	82 mg	1.5 mg
brussels sprouts, cooked	1 cup	669 mcg	2 mcg	97 mg	1.3 mg
cabbage, raw	1 cup	69 mcg	1 mcg	29 mg	1.5 mg
carrot	1 large	15,503 mcg	1 mcg	11 mg	0.7 mg
carrot juice	1 cup	12,559 mcg	1 mcg	20 mg	1.0 mg
cauliflower, raw	1 cup	12 mcg	1 mcg	46 mg	0.1 mg
garlic, raw	1 clove	0 mcg	0.4 mcg	0.9 mg	0.0 mg
kale, raw	1 cup	3,577 mcg	1 mcg	80 mg	0.5 mg
leeks, cooked	1 cup	31 mcg	1 mcg	4 mg	0.7 mg
mushrooms, raw	1 cup	0 mcg	8 mcg	2 mg	0.3 mg
onions, white, cooked	1 cup	0 mcg	1 mcg	11 mg	0.8 mg
potato, baked	1 medium	0 mcg	1 mcg	16 mg	0.1 mg
pumpkin, cooked	1 cup	31,908 mcg	1 mcg	10 mg	2.6 mg
red bell pepper, raw	1 cup	2,840 mcg	0.3 mcg	175 mg	0.7 mg
spinach, raw	1 cup	1,196 mcg	0.3 mcg	8 mg	0.8 mg
squash, acorn, cooked	1 cup	627 mcg	2 mcg	26 mg	1.6 mg
sweet potato, cooked	1 cup	26,184 mcg	1 mcg	49 mg	0.6 mg
tomato, raw*	1 medium	446 mcg	0.5 mcg	23 mg	1.1 mg
yam, orange, baked	1 cup	26,184 mcg	1 mcg	49 mg	0.6 mg

* rich in lycopene

Sources for tables 10 and 11: Dietary Reference Intakes for Calcium, Phosphorous, Magnesium, Vitamin D, and Fluoride (1997); Dietary Reference Intakes for Thiamin, Riboflavin, Niacin, Vitamin B$_6$, Folate, Vitamin B$_{12}$, Pantothenic Acid, Biotin, and Choline (1998); Dietary Reference Intakes for Vitamin C, Vitamin E, Selenium, and Carotenoids (2000); Dietary Reference Intakes for Vitamin A, Vitamin K, Arsenic, Boron, Chromium, Copper, Iodine, Iron, Manganese, Molybdenum, Nickel, Silicon, Vanadium, and Zinc (2001); and Dietary Reference Intakes for Water, Potassium, Sodium, Chloride, and Sulfate (2004). These reports may be accessed via *www.nap.edu*.

TABLE 12 Antioxidants in grains and grain products

GRAIN OR GRAIN PRODUCT	SERVING SIZE	BETA-CAROTENE	SELENIUM	VITAMIN C	VITAMIN E
barley, cooked	1 cup	0	36 mcg	0	3.0 mg
brown rice, cooked	1 cup	0	14 mcg	0	1.1 mg
millet, cooked	1 cup	0	2 mcg	0	1.3 mg
oatmeal, cooked	1 cup	0	19 mcg	0	0.2 mg
wheat germ	2 tablespoons	0	11.4 mcg	0	2.6 mg
whole wheat bread	1 slice	0	10 mcg	0	0.3 mg

TABLE 13 Antioxidants in fruits

FRUIT	SERVING SIZE	BETA-CAROTENE	SELENIUM	VITAMIN C	VITAMIN E
apple	1 medium	28 mcg	0.4 mcg	8 mg	0.9 mg
apricots	3 medium	1,635 mcg	0.4 mcg	10 mg	0.9 mg
banana	1 medium	57 mcg	1.3 mcg	11 mg	0.4 mg
blueberries	1 cup	87 mcg	1 mcg	19 mg	2.7 mg
cantaloupe	⅛ melon	1,325 mcg	0.3 mcg	29 mg	0.2 mg
cantaloupe	1 cup cubes	3,072 mcg	0.6 mcg	68 mg	0.5 mg
grapefruit*	1 cup sections	160 mcg	3 mcg	79 mg	0.6 mg
grapes	1 cup	54 mcg	0.2 mcg	4 mg	0.3 mg
guava	1 cup	750 mcg	1 mcg	303 mg	1.8 mg
kiwi	2 medium	164 mcg	0.6 mcg	114 mg	1.7 mg
mango	1 cup cubes	3,851 mcg	1 mcg	46 mg	1.8 mg
orange	1 medium	52 mcg	1 mcg	59 mg	0.4 mg
orange juice	1 cup	92 mcg	0.2 mcg	124 mg	0.5 mg
papaya	1 cup cubes	70 mcg	0.8 mcg	87 mg	1.6 mg
peach	1 medium	260 mcg	0.4 mcg	6 mg	1.0 mg
raspberries	1 cup	48 mcg	0.7 mcg	31 mg	0.6 mg
strawberries	1 cup	23 mcg	1 mcg	82 mg	0.4 mg
watermelon*	1 cup cubes	634 mcg	0.3 mcg	27 mg	0.4 mg

* rich in lycopene

TABLE 14 Antioxidants in beans and legumes

BEAN OR LEGUME	SERVING SIZE	BETA-CAROTENE	SELENIUM	VITAMIN C	VITAMIN E
black beans, cooked	1 cup	10 mcg	2 mcg	0 mg	1.0 mg
black-eyed peas, cooked	1 cup	20 mcg	4 mcg	1 mg	0.5 mg
chickpeas, cooked	1 cup	28 mcg	6 mcg	2 mg	2.0 mg
kidney beans, cooked	1 cup	3 mcg	2 mcg	2 mg	0.4 mg
lentils, cooked	1 cup	11 mcg	6 mcg	3 mg	1.2 mg
pinto beans, cooked	1 cup	2 mcg	12 mcg	4 mg	1.6 mg
soybeans, cooked	1 cup	10 mcg	13 mcg	3 mg	3.4 mg
split peas, cooked	1 cup	11 mcg	1 mcg	1 mg	1.6 mg
tofu, firm	1 cup	0 mcg	44 mcg	1 mg	0.1 mg
white beans, cooked	1 cup	0 mcg	2 mcg	0 mg	2.0 mg

TABLE 15 Antioxidants in nuts, seeds, and oils

NUT, SEED, OR OIL	SERVING SIZE	BETA-CAROTENE	SELENIUM	VITAMIN C	VITAMIN E
almonds, raw	½ oz., 2 tablespoons, 12 nuts	0 mcg	1 mcg	0 mg	3.8 mg
Brazil nuts, raw	½ oz., 2 tablespoons, 3 nuts	0 mcg	420 mcg	0 mg	1.0 mg
cashews, raw	½ oz., 2 tablespoons	0 mcg	2 mcg	0 mg	1.0 mg
flaxseeds	1 tablespoon	0 mcg	6 mcg	1 mg	0.1 mg
olive oil	1 teaspoon	0 mcg	0 mcg	0 mg	0.6 mg
peanuts, roasted	½ oz., 2 tablespoons, 17 nuts	0 mcg	1 mcg	0 mg	1.1 mg
sunflower seeds	1 tablespoon	3 mcg	5 mcg	0 mg	5.0 mg
walnuts, raw	½ oz., 2 tablespoons, 7 nuts	0 mcg	0.6 mcg	3 mg	0.4 mg

It should be noted that tests of garlic's ability to block cancer promotion have been carried out in cells, not in intact humans, so it remains to be established whether garlic can actually affect the course of cancer after diagnosis.

Most people think of fruits and vegetables when referring to phytochemicals and antioxidants; however, grains contain important cancer-fighting compounds too. Grains have a unique phytochemical composition that can survive digestion and reach the colon. This may help explain why grain consumption has been associated with lower colon cancer rates.[16]

Immune-Boosting Foods

If you were to look at a sample of your blood under a microscope, you would see an enormous number of red blood cells, whose job is to carry oxygen to your body tissues. Here and there among them are white blood cells of various kinds, and they are the key soldiers that make up your immune system. When abnormal cells arise in the body, it is the job of white blood cells to recognize and eliminate them.

Some white blood cells are able to engulf and destroy abnormal cells, such as viruses, bacteria, and other invaders, including cancer cells. Other white blood cells facilitate this process in various ways, for example, by producing *antibodies*, protein molecules that attach to foreign or abnormal cells and flag them for destruction.

The immune system is critically important in fighting cancer. Individual cancer cells can arise in all of us from time to time. Cancer cells can also break free from an existing tumor and spread to other parts of the body. If your immune system is vigilant, it recognizes and destroys cancer cells before they can take hold. Thus, strengthening the immune system is a key strategy in cancer prevention and survival.

Like soldiers anywhere, your immune cells fight more effectively when they are well nourished. Certain antioxidants that we mentioned previously have been shown to be immune boosters: beta-carotene, vitamin C, and vitamin E. In addition, the mineral zinc is essential for the development and function of white blood cells.

Zinc

The mineral zinc has been promoted for its cold-fighting abilities, and, indeed, it works. However, when it comes to zinc or any other mineral, you want neither too little nor too much, just as we saw with vitamin E.[17] Researchers in New Jersey discovered this fact accidentally.[18] They tested zinc's effects in a group of older men and women. Some were given zinc tablets, while others got placebo tablets that looked and tasted just like zinc. And to make sure that everyone was generally well-nourished, the researchers also asked the participants to take a daily multiple vitamin.

When the researchers later checked the group's immune function, they found, to their surprise, that *everyone* had an immune boost. You can guess why. The multiple vitamin apparently counteracted a variety of mild nutritional deficiencies, and that improved their immunity. However, the researchers had a second, more surprising, finding: The volunteers who were taking as little as 15 milligrams of zinc actually had *worse* immune function than those who got placebos. In other words, zinc is an essential nutrient and a helpful immune booster when ingested in minute quantities. But it is easy to go overboard, and excess zinc *interferes* with immune function. The recommended amount of zinc in the daily diet is 8 milligrams for adult women and 11 milligrams for adult men. Table 16 lists some good foods that will keep your zinc intake up where it should be, without going too high.

TABLE 16 Good food sources of zinc

FOOD	AMOUNT OF ZINC
1 serving of most breakfast cereals	3.75 mg
1 Yves Veggie Burger	9.2 mg
½ cup tempeh	1.3 mg
½ cup peas	0.8 mg
½ cup cooked chickpeas	1.3 mg
1 cup soymilk	0.9 mg
2 tablespoon tahini	1.4 mg
2 tablespoon wheat germ	2.3 mg

Foods that Interfere with Immunity

In contrast to these healthful immune boosters, some parts of the diet interfere with immunity. Fatty foods, in particular, impair your immune cells' ability to work. Researchers have fed fatty foods to volunteers, dripped fatty intravenous solutions into volunteers' bloodstreams, and mixed fats with cancer cells. In each case, immune strength is noticeably reduced.[19,20] Simply put, your white blood cells don't work very well in an oil slick. While many people avoid animal fats—which is a good idea—they give themselves free rein with vegetable oils. But when it comes to boosting immunity, you'll want to minimize *all* fats and oils. This includes fish oils. Several research studies have suggested that fish oils can interfere with immunity.[21,22]

Fatty foods probably affect white blood cells directly. But they also tend to cause weight gain, and that can further impair immune function.[23] Studies show that overweight individuals are at increased susceptibility to various infections and to certain forms of cancer, especially postmenopausal breast cancer.

Cholesterol also seems to interfere with immunity. In case you are confused about the difference between fat and cholesterol: Fat is visible as a yellow layer under a chicken skin or white streaks marbled through a cut of beef. Cholesterol, on the other hand, resides as tiny particles inside the cell membranes that surround each cell in an animal's body, and *it is primarily in the lean portion*. Essentially all animal products contain cholesterol, while plant products never do.

When researchers add cholesterol to white blood cells in the test tube, it clearly interferes with their ability to function. Because your liver makes all the cholesterol your body needs for normal function, there is no need for any cholesterol in the diet.

Vegetarian Diets and Immunity

Vegetarian diets are typically rich in vitamins. In addition, they are generally low in fat, and vegetarians who also avoid dairy products and eggs (vegans) have no cholesterol in their diets at all. Vegetarian diets also help people lose excess weight; overweight people switching to a vegetarian diet typically lose about 10 percent of their body weight. So, theoretically, vegetarian diets ought to boost immunity.

That theory was put to the test at the German Cancer Research Center. Researchers drew blood samples from a group of vegetarians and compared them to healthy nonvegetarians working at the research center. They separated out a particular type of white blood cell called a *natural killer cell*. As its name implies, this type of cell really does shoot first and ask questions later. Natural killer (or NK) cells engulf and destroy cancer cells. By mixing the volunteers' NK cells with standardized samples of cancer cells, the researchers found that the vegetarians had approximately double the natural killer cell activity compared to the nonvegetarians.[24]

Meal Planning

Here are some simple tips that will help you build generous amounts of antioxidants, phytochemicals, and immune-boosting foods into your diet:

- Include plenty of vegetables and fruits in your routine, emphasizing the colorful varieties. Shoot for at least seven servings per day. One serving of vegetables is one-half cup cooked or one cup raw. For fruit, a serving is one small whole fruit or one-half cup chopped fruit.

- Keep a bag of baby carrots (rich in beta-carotene) nearby. Try them plain or dipped in hummus or a light vinaigrette.

- Limit storage of fruits and vegetables. Once they are separated from the plant, their carotenoids begin to break down.

- Check out your local Asian or Latin American grocery store to discover some new vegetables. For fresh seasonal produce, check out your local farmers' market.

- Avoid overcooking vegetables. While you still get a substantial amount of antioxidants in cooked vegetables, you will get much more if you don't cook them. A few exceptions, such as carrots and tomatoes, actually release more carotenoids when they have been cooked. If you don't like cooked carrots, try finely chopping raw carrots to release more of their carotenoids.

- Have plenty of tomato products (rich in lycopene): Mix sun-dried tomatoes into bread dough or add them to a veggie sandwich. Top pasta with marinara sauce (and add frozen vegetables, such as chopped spinach or kale, to the sauce as it cooks). Add canned tomatoes or salsa to a bean burrito, or top a veggie burger with ketchup or salsa. Reach for tomato juice to quench your thirst. Or make a quick bruschetta by toasting baguette slices, and then topping them with canned diced tomatoes and a sprinkling of basil.

- Crush a Brazil nut (rich in selenium) on top of your vegetable salad.

- Enjoy beans and whole grains for vitamin E and selenium.

- Add blueberries (rich in vitamin E) to your cereal or fruit smoothie.

- Add barley (rich in vitamin E and selenium) instead of pasta to vegetable soups and stews.

- Add broccoli, cauliflower, or any other of the other cruciferous veggies to stir-fries, soups, stews, and sauces.

- Boost any salad's cancer-fighting potential by adding cabbage, collard greens, kale, or watercress.

- Use rutabagas or turnips in place of potatoes in your favorite potato dish.

- Add fresh garlic to almost any meal.
- Take a multiple vitamin each day.
- Build your diet from plant foods and stay away from animal products. By doing so, you'll avoid most fat and all dietary cholesterol to help keep your immune system operating at its best.
- Avoid added oils and you'll keep fat content very low and immunity high.

Recommended Recipes

Buckwheat Pasta with Seitan (page 189)
Spinach Salad with Citrus Fruit (page 148)
Zippy Yams and Collards (page 184)

To Do This Week

Prepare one meal rich in beta-carotene and another rich in lycopene. This is easy, of course—it is as simple as cooking up some carrots and pouring tomato sauce over your angel hair pasta.

Select your recipes and plan a time that is convenient for you to pick up the ingredients you'll need. When you enter the grocery store to pick up your ingredients, pause for a moment in the produce aisle. Notice the bright colors and the fact that the same colors tend to show up over and over. Which foods have beta-carotene's distinctive color? That's right—you see it in cantaloupes, sweet potatoes, carrots, and occasionally in other foods.

Which ones have lycopene? It just about jumps out of the tomato bins. And you'll see it in the big watermelon slices and pink grapefruit.

Look at chlorophyll's bright green color almost everywhere in the produce section, and all the various other intense colors. These pigments are not just there to look pretty in your shopping cart. They served to protect the plants, and they will protect you, too.

Also, try preparing any cruciferous vegetable that is new to you, or prepare an old favorite in a new way. For example, if brussels sprouts are new to you, try this: Start with frozen petite brussels sprouts—the smaller they are, the lighter the taste. Steam them until they are soft and tender, then splash on some soy sauce, apple cider vinegar, or balsamic vinegar. You will be amazed. Try the same sort of technique with broccoli, collard greens, or kale.

If you've never had Swiss chard, it's time to try this wonderful vegetable. A few minutes of steaming turns it into a delightfully tender side dish. Top it with lemon juice. You'll find that the tartness of lemon juice or apple cider vinegar cuts through the faintly bitter taste of many vegetables and makes them truly delectable.

Maintaining a Healthy Weight

Many studies have shown that slimmer people are less likely to develop cancer. Trimming excess weight may also improve survival after cancer has been diagnosed. Among women with breast cancer, at least seventeen different research studies have shown that those who are thinner tend to live longer and have less risk of recurrence.[1]

Researchers have not had to look hard to find reasons to explain this finding. It has long been known that body fat is like a factory producing estrogens (female sex hormones). Hormones produced in the adrenal glands (small organs above each kidney) travel through the bloodstream into body fat. There, fat cells convert these hormones into estrogens.[1] In turn, estrogens fuel breast cancer growth, as we learned in chapter 1.

That's not all. Both women and men who have more body fat tend to have less of a protein compound called *sex hormone-binding globulin* (SHBG) in their blood. SHBG's job is to bind estrogen and testosterone, keeping these hormones inactive and unable to promote cancer. If overweight people have less SHBG, it means that more of their hormones are not reined in. They travel freely in the bloodstream, increasing the risk that cancer will start or, if it has already started, will spread to other parts of the body.

Excess weight may also reduce immune defenses. Researchers have shown that overweight people are more likely to show other signs of flagging immunity, such as recurrent infections. Poor immune defenses could mean they are less able to combat cancer cells that may arise.[2]

Body fat is like an estrogen factory. Fat cells convert hormones into estrogens.

Trimming Down the Healthy Way

So, how do we slim down? The first key is to focus not on *how much* you eat, but on *what* you eat. It is natural for people seeking to lose weight to skip meals and eat tiny portions. But doing so over even a few weeks tends to slow down your body's calorie-burning speed, making it harder and

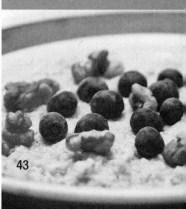

43

harder to lose weight. And cutting back on portions can make hunger get out of control, leading to binges and rebound weight gain.

Instead, focus on healthful foods that are naturally modest in calories. The best advice is to build your menu from the New Four Food Groups introduced in chapter 1. Vegetables, fruits, beans, and whole grains are nearly always lower in calories than typical meats, dairy products, eggs, and fried foods. This is partly because they are usually very low in fat. Ounce for ounce, fat has more than twice the calories of carbohydrate or protein. In addition, plant-based foods are so high in fiber, they tend to fill you up before you've taken in too many calories. Studies show that every 14 grams of fiber in our daily diet reduces our calorie intake by about 10 percent.[3]

By building your diet from the New Four Food Groups you'll avoid animal products and keep vegetable oils to an absolute minimum. In the process, you'll eliminate all animal fat and fiber-depleted foods and dramatically cut your fat intake. Several studies by the research team at the Physicians Committee for Responsible Medicine have shown that simply using the New Four Food Groups while avoiding animal products and keeping oils to a minimum leads to a weight loss of roughly one pound per week—week after week after week— *even if you don't exercise.* For example, in a study of fifty-nine postmenopausal women, the diet change caused participants to lose an average of thirteen pounds in fourteen weeks.[4] The same effect was seen in young women.[5] And in a study of individuals with type 2 diabetes, participants lost an average of thirteen pounds in just twenty-two weeks.[6] A recent review of eighty-seven studies on vegetarian or vegan diets and weight found that vegetarians were more likely to be at a healthy weight and that vegetarian diets brought greater weight loss than nonvegetarian diets.[7]

Studies show that every 14 grams of fiber in our daily diet reduces our calorie intake by about 10 percent.

Many other research studies have reached similar conclusions. You can focus on the type of food you eat—not the amount—and lose weight naturally and safely.

Of course, a slimmer body is not the only benefit of this type of nutritious menu. Low-fat vegetarian and vegan diets have been used to reverse heart disease, bring diabetes under control, lower blood pressure, reduce menstrual and premenstrual symptoms, and achieve many other health goals.[4-9]

Avoid Risky Diets

Some fad diets have had on-again, off-again popularity but are very detrimental over the long run. For example, low-carbohydrate, high-protein diets eliminate bread, pasta, beans, rice, starchy vegetables, and other carbohydrate-rich foods and focus instead on high consumption of meat and eggs. There are several things wrong with such diets.

First, controlled tests show that, over the long run, these diets cause no more weight loss than that associated with old-fashioned low-calorie diets or with nutritious low-fat vegan diets.

Second, when people lose weight with high-protein diets, it is simply because they are eliminating so many other foods that their overall calorie intake drops. If overall calorie intake doesn't drop, they don't lose weight.

Third, and most important, high-protein diets are linked to significant health problems.

Researchers have found that people on these diets lose large amounts of calcium in their urine, and the loss is caused by the massive amounts of protein they are consuming.[8] Animal protein tends to leach calcium from the bones and send it through the kidneys into the urine. Over the long run, that can lead to osteoporosis.

As we saw in chapter 4, meaty diets are linked to higher risk of colon cancer.[9,10] And high-fat diets in general are linked to poorer survival in individuals diagnosed with cancer.

For individuals battling serious illness—and for anyone else—it is a very good idea to lose excess weight, and it is important to do so in as healthful a way as possible.

Exercise

Exercise burns calories, boosts metabolism, and helps reduce the stresses that can lead to binge eating. But don't jump into a vigorous regimen too quickly. If you're over forty, significantly overweight, or dealing with any serious medical condition, you should check with your doctor before greatly increasing your physical activity.

When you start an exercise program, it pays to begin slowly. For most people, a brisk walk every day for half an hour—or three times per week for an hour—is a good way to begin.

If you are unable to exercise because of joint problems, cardiac limitations, or any other reason, you'll be glad to know that a low-fat diet based on the New Four Food Groups typically promotes weight loss even when people do not exercise. Yes, exercise is a good practice for lifelong health, but it is not essential for weight loss in particular.

Weight-Loss Keys

To summarize, here are the keys to healthy weight loss:

- Build your diet from the New Four Food Groups: vegetables, fruits, beans, and whole grains.
- Avoid animal products and added vegetable oils.
- Go high fiber, and enjoy plenty of vegetables, fruits, and bean dishes in as natural and unprocessed a state as possible. Choose high-fiber

grains, such as brown rice instead of white rice and whole-grain bread instead of white bread.

- Add any common multiple vitamin as a source of vitamin B_{12}.
- There are not many fatty plant foods, but it is good to minimize the ones there are—nuts, seeds, avocados, coconut, olives, and some soy products.
- If your doctor gives you the green light for regular physical activity, be sure to add exercise to your routine. Start slowly. Brisk walking for a half hour daily or an hour three times a week is a good way to begin. Then gradually increase your regimen.

Meal Planning

If you're aiming to knock off some pounds, this is a great time for a new focus on high-fiber foods. They tend to be very low in fat, so they won't add many calories. And they will fill you up, so you're less likely to overdo it.

If you were to include high-fiber foods at breakfast, lunch, and dinner, what would they be? Here are a few ideas; think about the ones that are most appealing to you:

Breakfast: Old-fashioned oatmeal is a natural choice. A bowl of strawberries, half a cantaloupe, or any seasonal fruit will add fiber, too. And, while it might sound a bit odd at first, a serving of chickpeas at breakfast provides plenty of protein and fiber, with very little fat. Try it; you'll like it. Whole-grain breads and bran cereals with low-fat soymilk or rice milk will also give you plenty of fiber.

Lunch: Start with salads loaded with fresh vegetables, beans, and low-fat salad dressing. For a hearty lunch, baked beans, lentil soup, or bean burritos are unbeatable. Or try hummus tucked into whole wheat pita bread with grated carrots, sprouts, and cucumbers, or spread low-fat black bean dip into a whole wheat tortilla and wrap it with peppers, tomatoes, and lettuce. A side of steamed green vegetables is always a great addition. And, if your tastes call for fresh fruit, a couple of pears or apples will give you loads of fiber with very few calories.

Dinner: For dinner, there are endless choices: vegetable stir-fry over brown rice, a chunky vegetable chili, lentil curry, vegetable fajitas loaded with fat-free refried beans and sautéed vegetables, or vegetable lasagne layered with tomato sauce, crumbled tofu, spinach, mushrooms, and cheesy-tasting nutritional yeast in place of the usual fatty meat and cheese. Or keep it simple and enjoy whole wheat pasta with a vegetable-rich marinara sauce. For dessert, try fresh fruit or a fruit sorbet.

Recommended Recipes

Blueberry Smoothie (page 100)   Rutabaga Mashed Potatoes (page 179)
Lentil Artichoke Stew (page 126)   Veggies in a Blanket (page 118)

Foods and Breast Cancer Survival

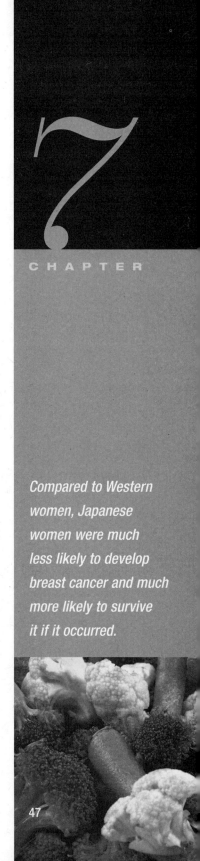

Healthful diets not only help prevent cancer, evidence suggests that they also improve survival when cancer has been diagnosed. The first clues that foods might affect the course of breast cancer came from studies of women in Japan in the early 1960s. Compared to Western women, Japanese women were much less likely to develop the disease and much more likely to survive it if it occurred.[1] Over the next several decades, researchers have followed up on these observations to try to clarify what is the best diet for cancer survival. Although this work is still in its early stages, important information has already come to light.

The Advantage of Being Thin or Losing Weight

One of the best-established factors affecting breast cancer survival is body weight. Women with breast cancer who are near their ideal body weight at the time of diagnosis are more likely to survive than are women with higher body weights. In a 2002 review of twenty-six studies published since 1990 on body weight and cancer recurrence or decreased survival in women previously diagnosed with breast cancer, seventeen studies showed that higher body weight was associated with increased risk; seven studies showed no relationship; and two showed an inverse relationship between body weight and risk.[2] Overall, the body of evidence supports a relationship between higher body weights and poor outcomes.

The relationship may hold even among relatively thin women. A 2006 study from Shanghai, China, studied the relationship between body mass index (BMI) and survival in 1,455 women aged twenty-five to sixty-four who had previously been diagnosed with breast cancer.[3] For reference, a healthy BMI is between 18.5 and 24.9 kg/m². Women with a BMI below 23 had a five-year survival rate of 86.5 percent. Those who were slightly heavier, with a BMI of 23.00–24.99, had a slightly lower five-year survival rate of 83.8 percent. Those with a BMI of 25 or greater had a five-year survival of 80.1 percent.

Compared to Western women, Japanese women were much less likely to develop breast cancer and much more likely to survive it if it occurred.

Although weight gain often occurs after diagnosis, studies suggest that women who avoid weight gain after diagnosis tend to have longer, disease-free survival.[2]

The link between lower body weight and better survival may relate to estrogens, female sex hormones that can encourage the growth of cancer cells. In essence, body fat acts like an estrogen factory, producing estrogens from other compounds coming from the adrenal glands (small organs situated atop each kidney). As a result, women with more body fat tend to have higher amounts of estrogens circulating in their blood compared to leaner women.

Reduced Fat Intake

Specific dietary factors appear to play key roles in cancer survival. First, two studies of women diagnosed with breast cancer showed that those who consumed less fat prior to diagnosis generally had smaller tumors with less evidence of cancer spread compared to women whose diets had included more fatty foods.[4,5] One of these studies identified benefits among pre-menopausal women and the other among postmenopausal women.

Studies that have followed women for several years after diagnosis have generally found that those with less fatty diets prior to diagnosis live longer than other women. In one of the first such studies, researchers at the State University of New York in Buffalo found that women with advanced cancer had a 40 percent increased risk of dying at any point in time for every 1,000 grams of fat they consumed per month.[6] Note that this does not mean a person's risk of dying is 40 percent. It means that if a person's diet contains an extra 1,000 grams of fat per month at the time of diagnosis, that person's risk of dying is 40 percent higher than it would otherwise have been. There is, of course, tremendous variation from one woman to another, so this figure is simply an overall observation drawn from the group of participants. To make this more concrete, the difference between a typical American diet and a low-fat vegan diet is approximately 1,000–1,500 grams of fat per month, which corresponds to a 40–60 percent difference in mortality risk at any point in time.

Other studies found much the same thing—fatty diets are associated with increased risk, and that is particularly true for saturated fat, the kind that is common in meat, dairy products, eggs, and chocolate.[7-10] Some studies have failed to confirm the dangers of fatty diets.[11-14] However, most evidence indicates that women consuming less fat tend to do better after diagnosis, including the Women's Intervention Nutrition Study (WINS), sponsored by the National Cancer Institute (NCI).[15] This study followed nearly 2,500 postmenopausal women with breast cancer for five years after their standard surgery and cancer treatments. Researchers instructed some of them to continue their regular diets while the rest were put on a low-fat diet. The women continuing their usual diets consumed an average of 51.3

grams of fat per day, which is still lower than the average American's fat, while the low-fat group averaged 33.3 grams per day—slightly more than in a typical vegetarian diet. After five years, 12.4 percent of the women eating their usual diet had cancer recurrences compared to only 9.8 percent of the low-fat diet group, a 24 percent reduction in recurrence.

Why does low fat intake improve survival? To begin with, low-fat diets tend to be modest in calories, since fats and oils are the densest source of calories of any food we consume. In fact, some investigators believe that the main problem with fatty diets is simply their high calorie content. In addition, women who eat less fat and more fiber tend to have less estrogen (independent of the difference in their body weight). They may also have stronger immune defenses that can help them fight cancer cells.

Evidence suggests that diet changes must be substantial to be effective. The Women's Health Initiative included 48,835 participants, aged fifty to seventy-nine, who were free of breast cancer, and tested a diet that emphasized vegetables, fruits, and grains.[16] Fat intake fell from 38 percent of calories at the beginning of the study to 24 percent at one year, but slipped back up to 29 percent at six years. After 8.1 years of follow-up, overall breast cancer risk fell 9 percent, but the difference was not statistically significant, meaning that it could have occurred due to chance. However, risk of one type of breast cancer—progesterone receptor-negative tumors—fell by 24 percent. While the study was not a survival study—it assessed the risk of cancer developing in the first place, rather than the course of the disease after diagnosis—it suggests that modest dietary changes may bring only modest results.

Increased Fiber

Fiber is essential to the body's ability to eliminate excess estrogens. As the liver filters estrogens from the blood, it sends them through the bile duct into the intestinal tract, where fiber soaks them up and carries them out of the body. A study in Sweden found that women with higher fiber intake at the time of breast cancer diagnosis were more likely to have smaller tumors compared to women with lower fiber intake.[17] The amount consumed was not particularly high. Those women with larger tumors (greater than 20 millimeters) averaged 16 grams of fiber per day compared to 19 grams for women with smaller tumors. Most authorities recommend fiber intake of at least 30 grams daily, and an optimal intake is probably over 40 grams.

Increased Vegetables and Fruits

Some evidence suggests that women whose diets are richer in vegetables and fruits tend to survive longer.[2,18] In a study of 103 women in Australia, who were followed for six years after they were diagnosed with breast cancer, those who consumed the most fruits and vegetables rich in beta-carotene or vitamin C had the best chance for survival. The researchers divided the group into thirds based on how much beta-carotene they got each day in the foods they chose. It turned out that in the group getting the least beta-carotene, there were twelve deaths over the next six years. In the middle group, there were eight deaths; and in the high-beta-carotene group, there was only one death.[19]

In the digestive tract, beta-carotene is converted to vitamin A. In turn, vitamin A is converted to a compound called *retinoic acid*, which has a demonstrable anticancer effect on cells in test-tube studies.[16] A Swedish study found much the same thing: Among women with breast cancer, those consuming more vitamin A were more likely to have estrogen receptor-rich tumors, a good prognostic sign.[17]

The Australian researchers also analyzed their data in another way, looking simply at how much fruit of any kind the women had been eating, including both beta-carotene-rich fruits and other varieties, such as apples, bananas, berries, grapes, and dried fruits. The same sort of pattern emerged. In the group eating the least fruit, there were twelve deaths; in the middle group, there were six deaths; and in the group consuming the most fruit, there were only three deaths.[19]

Similarly, a study of Canadian women with breast cancer found that those getting the most beta-carotene and vitamin C had significantly better survival odds.[9] The benefit was dose related, meaning the more of these helpful nutrients they got, the better they did. Those who got more than 5 milligrams of beta-carotene per day had double the likelihood of survival compared to women who got less than 2 milligrams. To understand what this means on your plate, there are about 5 milligrams of beta-carotene in half a medium carrot or one-fourth cup of cooked sweet potato.

For vitamin C, those getting more than 200 milligrams each day had roughly double the survival odds compared to those getting less than 100 milligrams per day. In practical terms, an orange has about 60 milligrams of vitamin C, and a one-cup serving of broccoli or other green vegetables has about 80.[9]

Vitamin E may have the opposite effect. In one study, women with breast cancer consuming larger amounts of vitamin E had poorer survival. Every one-milligram increase in daily vitamin E intake was associated with approximately a 15–20 percent increased risk of treatment failure.[8]

Combined Diet Effects: The Women's Healthy Eating and Living Study

These dietary factors tend to work together: A diet that is higher in fruits and vegetables will also tend to be high in fiber and low in fat. In turn, women who eat such diets tend to be slimmer than other women, thus avoiding the risks of overweight. One study suggested that there may be a measurable benefit of these combined effects. Researchers at Mt. Sinai Medical Center in New York found that women with breast cancer who were slimmer tended to live longer, and those who had lower cholesterol levels also lived longer. But the women at greatest risk of dying were those who were overweight and had high cholesterol levels.[20]

The Women's Healthy Eating and Living (WHEL) Study included more than 3,000 pre- and postmenopausal women previously treated for breast cancer in a test of two different diets rich in fruits and vegetables.[21] Half the participants (the intervention group) were asked to include in their daily diets five vegetable servings, 2 cups of vegetable juice, three fruit servings, 30 grams of dietary fiber, and no more than 15–20 percent of calories from fat. A comparison group was asked to consume at least five fruit and vegetable servings per day.

In 291 of the study participants, changes in diet and hormone function were compared between the two diet groups.[22] The women who ate less fat and more fiber found that the amount of estrogen in their blood fell to safer levels, confirming that diet changes really do help get hormones into better balance.

In the same study, the investigators tracked the experience of 1,551 women assigned to the comparison group, using blood tests for plasma carotenoids as an indicator of vegetable and fruit intake.[23] As in any large group, their diets varied from one person to another. It turned out that those with the highest carotenoid concentrations—indicating high vegetable and fruit intake—had a 43 percent lower risk of either cancer recurrence or a new primary breast cancer compared to women with lower blood levels of carotenoids.

After approximately seven years of follow-up, those women in the comparison group who followed the guideline of eating at least five fruit and vegetable servings daily and who were also physically active had an almost 50 percent reduction in mortality compared to women who did not meet these healthful guidelines.[24] However, the recommendations for even greater vegetable and fruit intake made for the intervention group did not extend benefits beyond those achieved by the five-a-day (comparison) group.[25]

While the WHEL participants succeeded at emphasizing vegetable and fruit intake, they did not maintain a low fat intake or a high fiber intake. The intervention group did reduce fat intake to 21 percent of calories in the first six months, but fat intake gradually climbed back to 29 percent by the six-year point. Similarly, fiber intake was only slightly higher at six years (24 grams per day) compared to the study's onset (21 grams). As a result, neither the intervention nor the comparison group succeeded at weight loss; both groups were overweight at the beginning of the study and gained a small amount of weight as the study progressed. A vegetarian or vegan regimen may have been a better choice; the meat and dairy products that were permitted in the WHEL guidelines contain significant amounts of fat and contribute no fiber.

Nonetheless, the WHEL study demonstrated that women previously treated for breast cancer who consume at least five vegetable and fruit servings daily and are physically active have a large measure of protection (nearly 50 percent reduction in mortality), and their protection is not increased by pushing vegetable intake even higher. The study did not test other potentially helpful dietary measures.

Exercise

Exercise may also improve breast cancer survival. A study published in the *Journal of the American Medical Association* concluded that physical activity after breast cancer diagnosis may reduce a woman's risk of death from the disease. In this study, the greatest benefit was shown in women who exercised the equivalent of walking at an average pace for three to five hours per week.[26]

Recommended Recipes

Berry Applesauce (page 214)
Broccoli or Cauliflower with Sesame Salt (page 174)
Home-Style Squash and Pinto Beans (page 192)
Hot or Cold Beet Salad (page 143)

Foods and Prostate Cancer Survival

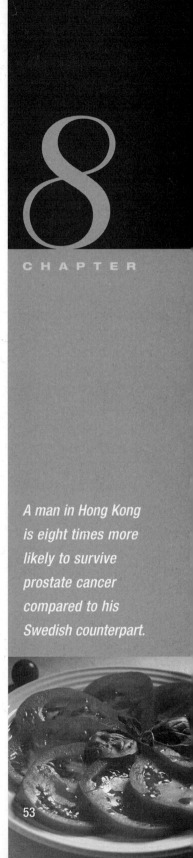

Many research studies have shown how foods affect the risk of developing prostate cancer. Vegetables and fruits reduce the risk, while dairy products and fatty foods appear to increase it.

But what about *after* prostate cancer has been diagnosed? Will a change in eating habits help beat the disease? More research is needed, but evidence already available suggests that, whatever other treatments a man may undergo, changes in his diet might well save his life.

The first clues that diet could make a big difference in survival emerged from international comparisons in the 1970s. A man in Hong Kong, where diets are rich in rice and vegetables, is half as likely to have cancerous cells in his prostate compared to a man in Sweden, where diets are high in dairy products and meat. But if cancer happens to strike, a man in Hong Kong is *eight times more likely to survive it* compared to his Swedish counterpart.[1] In other words, it appears that the same sort of dietary habits that reduce the risk of cancer also slow its progress if it occurs.

Why would dietary changes help? One explanation relates to *insulin-like growth factor 1* (IGF-1), a substance in the bloodstream that is a powerful stimulus for cancer cell growth. Men following plant-based diets have lower IGF-1 levels than other men, while dairy products tend to drive IGF-1 levels up. Men following low-fat, high-fiber diets also have slightly lower testosterone and estrogen levels and higher levels of a protein called *sex hormone-binding globulin*, which binds and temporarily inactivates testosterone and estrogen. The net effect is a drop in the biochemical factors that stimulate cancer growth.

A man in Hong Kong is eight times more likely to survive prostate cancer compared to his Swedish counterpart.

Putting Diet to the Test

The first prospective studies of diet's potential benefits were purely observational. In 1999, researchers in Québec City reported their findings after following 384 men with prostate cancer over a five-year period. It turned out that those who consumed the most saturated fat—the kind particularly prevalent in meats and dairy products—had three times the risk of dying from the disease compared to those with the lowest saturated fat intake. Increased risk was also found with higher intakes of total and monounsaturated fat, but these increases were not significant.[2]

The following year, researchers in Toronto and Vancouver reported the results of a study of 263 men with prostate cancer. The study found that the men who consumed the most monounsaturated fat (the type that is abundant in olive and canola oils) lived the longest. Their risk of dying was 70 percent lower compared to those with the lowest intake of monounsaturates. The study also found increased risk from animal fat and saturated fat intake, although these latter findings were not strong enough to reach statistical significance.[3]

Using a Vegan Diet

Dean Ornish, founder and director of the Preventive Medicine Research Institute and clinical professor of medicine at the University of California, San Francisco, who had already demonstrated the benefits of a low-fat, vegetarian diet for heart patients (finding that it reversed heart disease in 82 percent of research participants), decided to put a similar program to the test for prostate cancer.[4] The ninety-three volunteers were men with early-stage cancer who were able to defer treatment, at least for the moment, because they were keeping a careful watch on their prostate-specific antigen (PSA, an index of cancer spread) levels, a strategy known as "watchful waiting." Typically, PSA levels slowly rise, and eventually treatment (such as surgery) may be required. Ornish randomly assigned half of the men to follow their usual habits (the control group), and the remaining half were to follow a low-fat vegan diet along with moderate aerobic exercise and stress management. In the experimental vegan group, PSA levels decreased by 4 percent after one year, while PSA levels rose by 6 percent in the control group. Six of the men in the control group needed treatment during the one-year study period because their prostate cancer was progressing, whereas no one in the experimental group needed treatment during the study period.

Using Diet to Fight Recurrent Cancer

Ornish's approach is extremely promising for men with early prostate disease. But what about advanced cancer? Evidence suggests that dietary changes can still play a vital role. Two studies have used special diets in men who had previously been operated on for prostate cancer but who had experienced recurrences of their disease. Using a macrobiotic diet emphasizing whole grains, vegetables, and legumes, while avoiding dairy products and most meats, nine men with prostate cancer had an average survival of 228 months compared to 72 months for a matched group of men receiving no special diet.[5]

A study at the University of Massachusetts tested the benefits of a dietary change in ten men with prostate cancer that had recurred after surgery. The diet was based on whole grains, legumes, green and yellow vegetables, seeds, soy products, and fruit, and the men were also instructed in stress-reduction techniques. To measure the program's effect, researchers tracked how long it took for the patients' PSA levels to double—the longer the PSA doubling time, the slower the cancer is spreading. Before the study began, the average PSA doubling time was 6.5 months. But after four months in the program, it had slowed to 17.7 months, an encouraging finding. In three of the men, PSA levels actually fell.[6]

Cancer-Fighting Power You Can See

In 2002, researchers at the University of California at Los Angeles reported a series of unusual experiments that demonstrated the power of diet and exercise. They drew blood samples from a group of eight men who had been following a low-fat diet and exercising regularly for several years. They also drew blood samples from overweight men who were not following the diet and exercise program. They added portions of each man's blood serum to test tubes containing standardized prostate cancer cells. Serum from men on the low-fat diet and exercise program slowed cancer cell growth by 49 percent compared to serum from the other men. How could this be? Differences in testosterone, estrogen, and insulin account for part of the effect, but other changes in the blood exert additional effects the researchers have not yet teased out.[7] The research team also found that a man's serum shows demonstrable cancer-inhibiting power within as little as eleven days after beginning a low-fat diet and exercise regimen.[8]

Lycopene and Prostate Cancer

Part of the value of plant-based diets comes from the protective compounds they contain. As we saw in chapter 5, carotenoids are a specific class of antioxidants that includes lycopene, lutein, α-carotene and β-carotene. This class of antioxidants is primarily found in vegetables and fruits. Lycopene is considered one of the most potent antioxidants in the carotenoid family and has been linked with reduced prostate cancer risk.[9,10] The highest concentrations of lycopene are in cooked tomato products, such as pasta sauce. Smaller but significant amounts are also found in raw tomatoes, grapefruit, watermelon, and guava. A 2004 meta-analysis evaluating lycopene and prostate cancer risk concluded that high tomato and lycopene intake may reduce prostate cancer risk by 10–20 percent.[11] Diet intervention studies in newly diagnosed patients with localized prostate adenocarcinoma have found that consuming as little as 30 milligrams a day of lycopene in whole food or supplement form may reduce serum PSA levels.[12]

The Bottom Line

While more research will be of great value, evidence already suggests that men with prostate cancer—and their families—should be encouraged to adopt a low-fat vegan diet. By boosting vegetables, fruits, beans, and whole grains, and avoiding dairy products, meats, eggs, and fried foods, men are able to take advantage of protective nutrients and avoid cancer-promoting factors.

Recommended Recipes

Braised Kale (page 173)
Mushroom Gravy (page 156)
No-Meat Loaf (page 195)
Tomato, Cucumber, and Basil Salad (page 150)

Planning Health-Promoting Meals

You now have the basic knowledge and cooking skills you need to begin to make some major changes in your eating habits. There is much more to learn, of course, but now's the time to put what you know to work. In this chapter, you'll have a chance to experience what it is like to be on as perfect a diet as possible. We will use a unique method to learn new tastes and break away from bad habits. Along the way, we will also look at what to do when you do not have complete control over the menu, for example at restaurants or fast-food outlets.

The Three-Week Break

The best and easiest way to try a new way of eating is to take what you might call a "three-week break." That is, select a three-week period and during this time build your meals only from the best possible foods while setting aside unhealthful foods completely. Your taste buds have a memory of about three weeks, which means that, in that short time, you'll be adjusted to new tastes. So whether you are looking to cut the fat from your diet, reduce salt, break a sugar habit, or get to know truly health-promoting foods, using a three-week break—and really doing it all the way—will give you the momentum you need.

At the end of three weeks, see how you feel. If you like how things are going—if you've lost a few pounds and are feeling healthier and more energetic—you can stick with it. If, however, this just doesn't feel right to you, you are free to go back to your old way of eating. Your diet experiment lasts only three weeks, and remembering that will help you to give it your all.

Do not do it halfway. Now is the time to really see what healthful eating feels like. If you were just to have an occasional nutritious vegetarian meal while continuing to eat meaty, cheesy dishes at other times, you would keep reminding your taste buds of the very foods that cause health problems and would never lose your taste for these foods. Have a complete

The best and easiest way to try a new way of eating is to take what you might call a "three-week break."

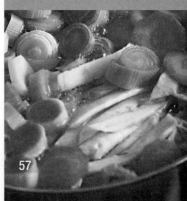

57

break and really try to eat only health-supporting foods. In chapter 3, we talked about the common experience of switching from whole milk to skim or nonfat versions to illustrate how quickly we adjust to lighter tastes. Well, now is your chance to lighten up your entire menu. At first, your taste buds might miss fatty foods, but that will soon pass as they come to embrace more wholesome choices.

Use the New Four Foods Groups

For cancer-fighting power, put the New Four Food Groups from chapter 1 into practice. Build your diet from whole grains, legumes, vegetables, and fruit, while avoiding animal products (meat, poultry, dairy products, and eggs) and fried foods (such as potato chips, french fries, onion rings, tempura, and donuts), and keeping vegetable oils and other high-fat plant foods to a minimum. If you like, you may use coffee and tea with soy creamers and low-fat vegan salad dressings and condiments, such as low-fat Italian dressing, ketchup, mustard, relish, soy sauce, tamari, and fat-free or low-fat vegan mayonnaise. Nuts and seeds should be treated as condiments rather than food groups, as they are high in fat.

The nutrition guidelines in table 17 and the corresponding checklist on page 63 will help you get started.

Protein

Eating a variety of plant foods will give you all the protein you need. The recommended intake of protein is approximately 10 percent of calories, or 0.8 grams for every kilogram of body weight. On a 2,000 calorie diet, 10 percent of calories equals 50 grams of protein. Or, using the body weight equation, an individual who weighs 150 pounds (68 kilograms) should be getting approximately 54 grams of protein per day. Most vegetables, legumes, and grains derive at least 10 percent of their calories from protein. Legumes and meat alternatives (such as tofu, seitan, and veggie burgers) are especially rich sources, with at least 20 percent of their calories coming from protein. For more information on protein and other nutrition fundamentals, see chapter 11, Nutrition Basics (page 85).

Calcium

There's plenty of highly absorbable calcium in dark leafy greens, such as bok choy, kale, mustard greens, collard greens, and turnip greens, as well as broccoli, legumes, figs, almonds, calcium-fortified juices, calcium-fortified soymilk, and rice, almond, and oat milks. These foods contain other cancer-fighting nutrients that are not present in dairy products. For more information on bone health and the calcium content of plant foods, see chapter 3, Discovering Dairy Alternatives (page 17).

TABLE 17 Serving sizes and food examples for the New Four Food Groups

FOOD GROUP	RECOMMENDED DAILY SERVINGS	SUGGESTED SERVING SIZE	FOOD EXAMPLES		
fruits	3+ servings	1 small fruit ½ cup berries or chopped fruit ½ cup unsweetened fruit juice	apples bananas blueberries citrus fruits	grapes kiwi mangoes melon	peaches pears strawberries
legumes	3+ servings	1 cup nondairy milk ½ cup cooked beans ¼ cup low-fat bean spread 3 ounces soy products or meat alternative	baked beans black beans chickpeas kidney beans	lentils rice milk seitan soybeans	soymilk tempeh tofu veggie burgers
vegetables	4+ servings	1 cup colorful raw vegetables ½ cup colorful cooked vegetables	artichokes bok choy broccoli cauliflower	collard greens cucumbers green beans kale	spinach squash sweet potatoes tomatoes

whole grains	6+ servings	½ cup cooked grain
		¾–1 cup dry cereal
		1 slice whole-grain bread
		½ pita bread
		½ tortilla
		¼ bagel
			barley
			bran cereals
			brown rice
			bulgur wheat
				couscous
				millet
				oatmeal
					pumpernickel
					  or rye bread
					whole-grain
					  pasta

Vitamin B$_{12}$

The only nutrient missing in a completely plant-based diet is vitamin B$_{12}$. Vitamin B$_{12}$ is made by bacteria and needed in minute amounts in the diet. It is plentiful in fortified commercial cereals, fortified milk alternatives, some veggie burgers, and certain brands of nutritional yeast. Vitamin B$_{12}$ is also present in any common multivitamin. Check the labels for the words "cyanocobalamin" or "vitamin B12."

Sample Meals

Many of these foods may already be a part of your diet.

BREAKFAST

- cold cereals, such as bran flakes, with low-fat soymilk or rice milk and/or berries, peaches, or bananas

- hot cereals, such as oatmeal or hot whole-grain cereal, with nondairy milk, cinnamon, raisins, and/or applesauce
- low-fat meat alternatives, such as fat-free vegan sausage and vegan Canadian bacon
- melon, cantaloupe, bananas, or any other fruit
- oven-baked home fries, solo or smothered with mushrooms, peppers, and onions (sautéed in water or vegetable broth)
- various fruit smoothies
- whole-grain or pumpernickel toast topped with jam

Try these recipes for breakfast:

- Banana-Oat Pancakes (page 91)
- Breakfast Scramble (page 93)
- Fruited Breakfast Quinoa (page 94)
- Tofu French Toast (page 95)

LUNCH

Whether you dine in or out at lunchtime, there are many healthful and delicious options from which to choose. Here are some ideas to get you started.

Salads
- bean-based salads: three-bean, chickpea, lentil, or black bean and corn salads
- garden salad with low-fat dressing
- grain-based salads: noodle, couscous, bulgur, or rice salads

Soups
- legume-based soups: black bean, vegetarian chili, spinach lentil, minestrone, or split pea
- low-fat instant or prepared vegan soups
- vegetable-based soups: potato-leek, carrot-ginger, mixed vegetable, or mushroom-barley

Sandwiches and Wraps
- black bean and sweet potato burrito with corn and tomatoes
- black bean dip, peppers, tomatoes, and lettuce wrapped in a whole wheat tortilla
- CLT: cucumber, lettuce, and tomato sandwich with Dijon mustard
- hummus spread tucked into whole wheat pita with grated carrots, sprouts, and cucumbers
- Italian eggplant submarine sandwich: baked eggplant slices, pizza sauce, and mushrooms (sautéed in water or vegetable broth) on a whole-grain submarine sandwich roll

- sandwich made with low-fat meat alternatives, such as barbecued seitan
- vegan deli meat slices with your favorite sandwich veggies

Try these recipes for lunch:

- Asian Fusion Salad (page 135)
- Black Bean Chili (page 121)
- Creamy Root Soup (page 123)
- Easy Bean Salad (page 140)
- Eggless Salad Sandwich (page 203)
- Fiesta Salad (page 141)
- Roasted Red Pepper Hummus (page 113)
- Lentil and Bulgur Salad (page 144)
- Lentil Artichoke Stew (page 126)
- Red Bean Wraps (page 209)

DINNER IDEAS

Emphasize vegetables and grains in all your meals. For many, the evening meal is a good place to try new items. Typically, you might start with some beans, brown rice, or another whole-grain dish and add a serving or two of vegetables.

Whole Grains

- barley
- brown rice
- millet
- quinoa
- whole-grain bread
- whole-grain pasta
- whole-grain couscous

Vegetables

- broccoli, cabbage, cauliflower
- corn (note: corn is technically a grain, but it also works as a vegetable)
- greens (such as bok choy, broccoli, collard greens, kale, spinach, and Swiss chard), steamed and topped with soy sauce
- sweet potatoes: baked or mashed, topped with steamed vegetables, salsa, Dijon mustard, black pepper, or black beans

Legumes

- baked beans
- black beans, chickpeas, kidney beans, pinto beans
- lentils, split peas
- vegetarian refried beans

Main Dishes

- beans and rice: try black beans with salsa, vegetarian baked beans, or fat-free refried beans with brown rice
- chili: low-fat homemade or canned chili or vegetarian boxed mixes
- fajitas made with sliced bell peppers, onion, and eggplant (sautéed in water or vegetable broth) and fajita seasonings, then stuffed into whole-grain tortillas
- low-fat vegetarian burgers served on whole-grain rolls with sliced veggies
- rice pilaf, Spanish rice, or vegan packaged rice dinners, with added beans and vegetables
- soft tacos: use whole-grain flour or corn tortillas and stuff them with beans, lettuce, tomato, and salsa
- veggie lasagne made with low-fat tofu (to replace the ricotta) and layered with grilled veggies
- whole-grain pasta with marinara sauce: if using a commercially prepared sauce, check to make sure it is low in fat and does not contain cheese

Try these recipes for dinner:

- Black Bean Chili (page 121)
- Chickpea Burgers (page 204)
- Lazy Lasagne (page 193)

DESSERTS

- fresh, dried, or cooked fruit
- fresh fruit sorbets

Try these recipes for dessert:

- Ambrosia (page 213)
- Berry Applesauce (page 214)
- Harvest Pudding (page 219)
- Summer Fruit Compote (page 222)

SNACKS

- bran cereal with soymilk
- carrot or celery sticks
- dried fruit
- fresh fruit
- hummus on whole wheat pita
- pumpernickel or rye toast with jam
- vegetarian instant soups (black bean, lentil, split pea, etc.)

The Daily Diet Checklist

The following food guide will provide you with approximately 1,200 calories. Additional servings in any of the groups can be added to provide more food throughout the day as long as the minimum number of servings is met. Photocopy this page and check off your daily servings.

FOOD GROUP	MINIMUM SERVING RECOMMENDATIONS
FRUIT (one serving = 80 calories)	Aim for 3 servings of fruit each day. A serving is ½ cup chopped fruit or berries or 1 small piece of fruit. Include nutrient-dense fruits, such as strawberries, blueberries, and citrus fruits. *Check off the servings:* ☐ ☐ ☐
LEGUMES (one serving = about 100 calories)	Aim for at least 3 servings of legumes each day. A serving is ½ cup cooked beans, ¼ cup low-fat bean spread, 1 cup nondairy milk, or 3 ounces tofu, tempeh, seitan, or meat alternative. *Note:* Some cancer patients avoid soy products. Other beans, lentils, seitan, rice milk, oat milk, and almond milk are nutritious choices in this group. *Check off the servings:* ☐ ☐ ☐
VEGETABLES (one serving = 35–50 calories)	Aim for at least 4 servings of vegetables each day. A serving equals ½ cup cooked or 1 cup raw vegetables. Choose a colorful variety each day to ensure that you get an array of cancer-fighting antioxidants. *Check off the servings:* ☐ ☐ ☐ ☐
WHOLE GRAINS (one serving = about 80 calories)	Aim for at least 6 servings each day and choose *whole* grains whenever possible. A serving is ½ cup cooked grain (such as oatmeal or pasta), 1 ounce dry cereal (usually ¾–1 cup), 1 slice of bread, or half a pita bread or tortilla. A bagel is considered 4 servings. *Check off the servings:* ☐ ☐ ☐ ☐ ☐ ☐

TABLE 18 Pesticide levels in fruits and vegetables

LOWEST PESTICIDE LEVELS			HIGHEST PESTICIDE LEVELS		
asparagus	cauliflower	papaya	apples	imported grapes	potatoes
avocados	kiwi	pineapples	bell peppers	nectarines	red raspberries
bananas	mangoes	sweet corn	celery	peaches	spinach
broccoli	onions	sweet peas	cherries	pears	strawberries

Source: Environmental Working Group, "A shopper's guide to pesticides in produce," October 27, 2005.

Go Organic

For better nutrition, choose organic, locally grown foods whenever possible to avoid potentially carcinogenic pesticides and fertilizers. If a completely organic diet is not available or affordable, you can prioritize your choices. The information in table 18 is courtesy of the Environmental Working Group. This table lists the twelve fruits and vegetables with the highest and lowest pesticide levels.

Making It Work

A note of caution: Merely *resolving* to eat right doesn't work very well. It's too easy to slip off track. To make sure it really does work for you, you need to do a few things:

First, *plan* what you will eat. Use the form on page 65 or any handy sheet of paper (yes, really do it) and mark down "breakfasts," "lunches," and "dinners." Under each heading, list foods that meet the New Four Food Groups guidelines and that work for you.

Second, *go out and buy* these foods so they're in your kitchen when you need them.

Third, and most important, *throw away everything else.* If you're threatened by a serious illness, health-damaging foods are not your friends. Get rid of them.

Okay, let's get started. If you're testing out new recipes, expect that some will turn out better than you anticipate and some might have the opposite result. Don't worry. That's what experimenting is all about.

Meal Planning Tips

Explore new recipes, new books, and new vegan foods as you become familiar with the New Four Food Groups. Low-fat meat and dairy alternatives, such as veggie burgers, soy-based or other mock meats, soy yogurts, or rice cheese, can speed the transition from an omnivorous diet to a plant-based regimen. To help cut the fat out of your meals, top potatoes with baked beans, black pepper, Dijon mustard, hot sauce, Italian seasoning, or

Meal Planning

BREAKFASTS

_____
_____
_____
_____
_____

LUNCHES

_____
_____
_____
_____
_____

DINNERS

_____
_____
_____
_____
_____

salsa, and steam or sauté vegetables in water or vegetable broth instead of oil or, rarely, use vegetable oil spray.

When you're on the go, bring low-fat snacks or a bag lunch in case wholesome foods are not readily available. Good convenience foods are bagels, low-fat granola bars, hummus and veggie pita sandwiches, fresh fruit, dried fruit, pretzels, crackers with bean spread, and instant bean or vegetable soups. While traveling, request vegan meals on flights and bring snacks along as well. Most hotels have fruit, oatmeal, pasta with tomato sauce, potatoes, and vegetable plates. Instant soups and instant oatmeal are easy to bring on trips and may come in handy.

Grocery Shopping

Shopping for healthful food doesn't have to be overwhelming if you know where to look. Use table 19 to help navigate your way to health-promoting food in the different sections of the grocery store.

TABLE 19 What to look for in the grocery store

AISLE	BEST CHOICES	FOOD EXAMPLES	
bakery	breads that list "whole wheat" or "bran" as the first ingredient; look for those without additives or preservatives	corn and flour tortillas pita bread whole wheat or pumpernickel bagels whole wheat pizza crust	
canned goods	beans fruits packed in juice or light syrup low-fat bean and vegetable soups low-sodium vegetables	bean soup beets black-eyed peas chickpeas corn kidney beans lentil soup	lentils minestrone navy beans peaches pineapple vegetable soup
dry goods	dried beans low-fat soup mixes nondairy milks in aseptic cartons whole grains whole-grain crackers whole-grain pasta	almond milk baked brown rice crackers bran cereal brown rice (regular and quick-cooking) brown rice spaghetti dried lentils rice milk	rolled oats soymilk split peas whole wheat pasta whole-grain mixes wild rice (regular and quick-cooking)
frozen foods	berries fruits single-serving and family-size meals vegetables and vegetable combinations veggie burgers whole-grain bread products	blueberries broccoli fruit combinations grilled veggie burgers mango chunks spinach vegan bean burritos	vegetable combinations whole-grain bagels whole-grain waffles whole wheat pita whole wheat pizza shells
produce	colorful and seasonal fresh fruits and vegetables	bananas bell peppers blueberries broccoli carrots	kale peaches pears strawberries yams
refrigerator case	bean dips and spreads bean salads low-fat vegetable salads meat alternatives nondairy milks nondairy yogurt tempeh tofu	baked or smoked tofu barbecued tempeh black bean dip hummus	soy yogurt tabouleh tofu salad vegan deli meat slices

Revising Conventional Recipes

Deciding to choose more healthful foods doesn't mean you can't still enjoy Grandma's famous cream of mushroom soup. Most recipes can be easily modified to be health-supporting and still remain delicious. Use the substitutions in table 20 when you are revising recipes.

TABLE 20 Replacing ingredients in conventional recipes

INSTEAD OF THESE INGREDIENTS	USE THESE ALTERNATIVES	TIPS
butter and oil in baked goods	<ul><li>applesauce</li><li>prune paste</li><li>soymilk</li></ul>	some fat alternatives will change the taste or texture of the finished product
butter and oil in cooking	<ul><li>vegetable broth</li><li>water</li></ul>	sauté vegetables in vegetable broth to add flavor without adding fat
cow's milk	<ul><li>almond milk</li><li>oat milk</li><li>rice milk</li><li>soymilk</li></ul>	for soups and savory dishes, always purchase plain or unsweetened nondairy milk
cream	<ul><li>blended silken tofu</li><li>blended white beans</li><li>mashed potatoes</li></ul>	make thick, creamy soups by blending in white beans, potatoes, or silken tofu
eggs as binders in burgers and loaves	<ul><li>mashed potatoes</li><li>moistened bread crumbs</li><li>rolled oats</li><li>tomato paste</li></ul>	tomato paste may change the color or taste of the finished product
eggs in baked goods	for each egg use one of the following:<ul><li>1 heaping tablespoon soy flour or cornstarch plus 2 tablespoons water</li><li>1 ounce mashed tofu</li><li>½ mashed banana</li><li>powdered egg-free egg replacer as per the package directions</li></ul>	<ul><li>if a recipe calls for only 1 or 2 eggs, you can often just omit them; add 1–2 extra tablespoons of water for each egg eliminated to balance out the moisture content</li><li>adding banana to baked goods may change the flavor of the finished product</li></ul>
meat, poultry, or fish	<ul><li>beans</li><li>eggplant</li><li>extra-firm tofu</li><li>portobello mushrooms</li><li>seitan</li><li>tempeh</li><li>vegan meat alternatives</li><li>veggie ground round</li></ul>	<ul><li>grilled portobello mushrooms make excellent burgers</li><li>vegan alternatives can replace meat products ounce for ounce in most recipes</li></ul>
sour cream and cream cheese	<ul><li>blended silken tofu</li><li>soy cream cheese</li><li>soy sour cream</li></ul>	make low-fat creamy dips, dressings, and desserts with blended silken tofu

Restaurants and Fast Food

More and more of our meals are served at restaurants, and much of what's on the menu is far from healthful. But that doesn't mean you have to forgo dining out. If you're a choosy about which restaurants you patronize and about what you order when you arrive, you'll still find plenty of great options.

For starters, it helps to think in terms of international foods. Restaurants that feature the cuisine of other lands often have a broad range of healthful menu items. For example, at an Italian restaurant you'll find minestrone, pasta and bean soup, pasta with marinara sauce, and green vegetables sautéed with garlic. Chinese and Thai restaurants have plenty of savory soups as well as vegetable-based main dishes featuring tofu, broccoli, green beans, spinach, and other nutritious ingredients. You'll also find a great many rice and noodle dishes. Ask them to use their more traditional cooking methods, without the added oil that may Westerners have come to expect. Japanese restaurants serve miso soup, salads, tofu, and vegetable sushi, all of which are usually very low in fat and delicately prepared.

Mexican restaurants serve hearty bean burritos, which, if prepared without lard and not smothered in cheese and sour cream, are usually low in fat and free of cholesterol. Indian restaurants always feature many delicious vegetarian choices, from appetizers to desserts. Ask the waiter to skip the dairy products and to be careful about the overzealous use of oil.

At generic restaurants and American steak houses, you'll find salad bars and vegetable plates. More and more fast-food and family-style restaurants are featuring veggie burgers, salad bars, and baked potato bars.

If you find yourself at a restaurant that does not have any health-supporting options on the menu, ask your server if the chef can prepare a vegetarian meal that does not include dairy products. Common examples include spaghetti with marinara sauce, a vegetable stir-fry over rice, or a baked potato with grilled vegetables. Chances are the kitchen has plenty of ingredients to prepare a wonderful vegan dish. And, since restaurants want their customers to leave happy, they should be more than willing to oblige.

Questions and Answers

ABOUT FOODS AND CANCER PREVENTION AND SURVIVAL

Alcohol

QUESTION: *How much alcohol is safe to consume?*

ANSWER: Although we occasionally hear of the reputed benefits of moderate alcohol consumption for reducing heart disease risk, even one drink per day, if consumed every day, increases breast cancer risk.[1] A recent review of alcohol consumption and cancer risk also showed increased risk for liver and colorectal cancer.[2]

Possible mechanisms by which alcohol may exert its cancer-causing effects include the toxic effect of alcohol metabolites, the production of free radicals, and disruption of folic acid's protective mechanisms. Polycyclic aromatic hydrocarbons, which are known carcinogens, have also been found in alcoholic beverages. In addition, alcohol consumption may lead to nutritional deficiencies, affecting the absorption of cancer-fighting nutrients.

Caffeine

QUESTION: *Does drinking coffee or other caffeinated beverages increase cancer risk?*

ANSWER: Probably not. Interest in this topic persists because coffee is such a popular beverage. In early 2006, a study suggested that coffee is responsible for as much as one-third of daily consumption of the cancer-causing chemical acrylamide, possibly as a result of the roasting of coffee beans. Earlier studies linked coffee consumption to increased risks of bladder and pancreatic cancers and a decreased risk of colon cancer.[3] Subsequent studies have not supported the link to pancreatic cancer. In addition, cigarettes may be the real culprit in the link between coffee consumption and bladder cancer, since smokers generally drink more coffee compared to the average consumer.[4] Studies on colon cancer, while mixed, lean toward a possible protective effect from coffee.[5]

Even one alcoholic drink per day, if consumed every day, increases breast cancer risk.

69

Regarding breast cancer, there is no evidence linking coffee consumption to an increased risk. However, caffeine may increase symptoms of fibrocystic breast disease, a common but benign breast condition.

According to a 2007 report by the American Institute for Cancer Research, a part of the World Cancer Research Fund global network, "Most evidence on coffee suggests that coffee drinking has no relationship with cancer risk."[6]

For bone health, heavy coffee use may be a problem. Excess caffeine consumption causes calcium to be leached from bones and excreted in the urine. Caffeine can also increase the heart rate, a concern in individuals with certain types of cardiac arrhythmias.

Calcium

QUESTION: *How much calcium is absorbed from plant foods?*

ANSWER: Table 21 lists the absorption percentages for calcium-rich plant foods. For comparison, 32 percent of the calcium from cow's milk is absorbed. Calcium-rich plant foods also contain many cancer-fighting nutrients that are not present in dairy products.

QUESTION: *How much calcium should a person get per day?*

ANSWER: Scientific evidence suggests that calcium intake should be at least 500–600 milligrams per day. Evidence of benefit from higher intakes is poor. It also makes sense to get plenty of exercise and to have about fifteen minutes of sunlight exposure daily to ensure adequate vitamin D.

TABLE 21 Absorption rate for calcium-rich plant foods

FOOD SOURCES	CALCIUM ABSORPTION PERCENTAGE
beans, white	17%
broccoli	52%
brussels sprouts	63%
kale	58%
mustard greens	57%
orange juice, calcium-fortified	37%
soymilk, calcium-fortified	24%
tofu, calcium-set	31%
turnip greens	51%

Sources: Weaver C. M., W. R. Proulx, and R. Heaney. Choices for achieving adequate dietary calcium with a vegetarian diet. *Am J Clin Nutr.* 1999;70(suppl):543S–548S. • Weaver C. M., and K. L. Plawecki. Dietary calcium: adequacy of a vegetarian diet. *Am J Clin Nutr.* 1994;59(suppl):1238S–1241S. • Keller J. L., A. J. Lanou, and N. D. Barnard. The consumer cost of calcium from food and supplements. *J Am Diet Assoc.* 2002;102:1669–1671.

One reason for being cautious about higher calcium intakes is that epidemiologic studies have linked high calcium intakes to an increased risk of prostate cancer. Good calcium sources include beans, figs, sweet potatoes, and especially dark green leafy vegetables, such as broccoli, collard greens, kale, mustard greens, and Swiss chard. Fortified soymilk and rice milk and calcium-fortified juices provide a great deal of calcium as well. It is also important to avoid calcium depleters—smoking, animal protein, excess sodium, and excess caffeine. In addition, eating lots of fruits and vegetables, excluding animal proteins, and limiting salt intake all help the body retain calcium.[7,8]

Childhood and Adolescence

QUESTION: *Does a vegan diet provide adequate nutrition for growing children?*

ANSWER: Yes. It is important to remember that eating habits are set in early childhood. Choosing a vegetarian diet can give your child—and your whole family—the opportunity to learn to enjoy a variety of nutritious foods. Children raised on vegetables, fruits, whole grains, and legumes grow up slimmer and healthier, and they live longer than their meat-eating friends. It is, in fact, much easier to build a nutritious diet from plant foods than from animal products, which contain saturated fat, cholesterol, and other substances that growing children can do without. As for essential nutrients, plant foods are the preferred source for children's diets, because they provide sufficient energy and protein packaged with other health-promoting nutrients, such as fiber, antioxidant vitamins, minerals, and phytochemicals.

Naturally, children need protein to grow, but they do not need high-protein, animal-based foods. A varied menu of grains, beans, vegetables, and fruits supplies plenty of protein. The "protein deficiencies" that our parents worried about in impoverished countries were the result of starvation or diets restricted to very few food items. Protein deficiency is extremely unlikely on a diet drawn from a variety of plant foods.

Very young children may need a slightly higher fat intake than adults do. In moderation, healthful fat sources include soybean products, avocados, and nut butters. Soy dogs, peanut butter and jelly sandwiches, seasoned veggie burgers, and avocado chunks in salads, for example, are very well accepted by children. However, the need for fat in the diet should not be taken too far. American children often have fatty streaks in their arteries—the beginnings of heart disease—before they finish high school. In contrast, Japanese children, who traditionally grow up on diets much lower in fat, subsequently have fewer problems with diabetes, heart disease, obesity, and other chronic diseases.

Parents will want to make sure their child's diet includes a regular source of vitamin B_{12}, which is needed for healthy blood and nerve function. Deficiencies are rare, but when they happen, they can be a bit hard to detect. Vitamin B_{12} is plentiful in many commercial cereals, fortified rice milk and soymilk, and some brands of nutritional yeast. Check the labels for the words "cyanocobalamin" or "B$_{12}$." It is strongly advisable for all children to take a daily multiple vitamin; it will provide adequate B$_{12}$. An alternative is to take a B$_{12}$ supplement of 5 micrograms or more per day. Spirulina and sea vegetables are not reliable sources of vitamin B$_{12}$.

The body also requires vitamin D, which is normally produced by sun on the skin. Exposing the hands and face to sunlight for fifteen to twenty minutes daily is usually enough for the body's skin cells to produce the necessary vitamin D. Children in latitudes with diminished sunlight may need the vitamin D found in multivitamin supplements or fortified nondairy milks.

Calcium is also an essential nutrient. Good calcium sources include beans and green vegetables, such as bok choy, broccoli, collard greens, kale, and mustard greens, and as well as dried figs and sweet potatoes. Fortified soymilk, rice milk, almond milk, or oat milk and calcium-fortified juices provide a great deal of calcium as well. In addition, eating lots of fruits and vegetables, excluding animal proteins, and limiting salt intake all help the body retain calcium.

Growing children also need iron, which is found in a variety of beans and green leafy vegetables. The vitamin C in vegetables and fruits enhances iron absorption when these foods are eaten along with an iron-rich food. One example is an iron-rich bean burrito eaten with vitamin C–rich tomato salsa. Few people are aware that cow's milk is very low in iron. It also reduces iron absorption and can induce mild, chronic blood loss in the digestive tract, which can reduce iron and cause an increased risk of anemia.

QUESTION: *How important is nutrition for young girls in families with a history of breast cancer?*

ANSWER: The foods girls eat while in preschool and grade school appear to have an important effect on breast cancer risk later in life. Researchers at Harvard University discovered that girls who eat more protein from animal sources and less protein from plant sources tend to reach menarche earlier.[9] Younger age at first menstruation is connected with increased risk of breast cancer later in life.[10] In addition, diet during puberty—while breast tissue is forming—also seems to have a significant influence on breast cancer risk in adulthood. Plant-based diets right from the start not only establish life-long smart eating habits, but also appear to be helpful in reducing breast cancer risk.

Cooking Food

QUESTION: *Does cooking destroy the cancer-fighting compounds in vegetables?*

ANSWER: For the most part, no. In a 2004 medical research review evaluating the effect of raw and cooked vegetables on cancer risk, both raw and cooked vegetables were related to reduced cancer risk.

Water-soluble nutrients, such as vitamin C and B vitamins, do tend to seep out of foods during boiling or steaming. However, if you reuse the cooking liquid in soups or to cook grains, you will get all the nutrients that have seeped out of the vegetables.

On the other hand, some antioxidants are actually released or activated by cooking, including the lycopene in tomatoes and the beta-carotene in carrots and sweet potatoes. Researchers have found that you can multiply the antioxidant power of carrots by cooking and puréeing them before eating. It turns out that cooking and puréeing releases cancer-fighting compounds from the carrot cells. To reap the full cancer-fighting benefits from the carrots you prepare, wash them thoroughly but avoid peeling them, as the skins are rich with cancer-fighting compounds.[11]

QUESTION: *What is the safest cookware?*

ANSWER: Various types of cookware have pros and cons. It is important that all cookware be replaced when dented or worn. If you see any chipping, throw it out.

- **Stainless steel**. Stainless steel is really a mixture of several different metals, including nickel, chromium, and molybdenum, all of which can leach into foods if your cookware is nicked or damaged. However if you take care of your pots and pans, this is probably one of the safest choices for cookware.
- **Cast iron**. Cast iron can help ensure that you are getting enough iron, as it is transferred from the cookware into food in small amounts. In large quantities, however, iron becomes a pro-oxidant, causing stress and oxidation in the body that can lead to disease. Most cast-iron pans need to be seasoned with oil after use.
- **Teflon**. It is important not to leave Teflon cookware on a burner or in a hot oven without liquid; this will release a chemical toxin called perfluorooctanoic acid (PFOA). Studies show that this chemical can be released when Teflon cookware is heated to as low as 464 degrees F.[12,13]
- **Aluminum**. Aluminum contact should be limited or avoided as much as possible, because of its possible link with Alzheimer's disease and its potential of having estrogen-like effects in the body. Anodized aluminum cookware is a safer alternative.[14]

Cost

QUESTION: *Doesn't healthful eating cost more?*

ANSWER: Surprisingly, choosing health-promoting foods over high-fat and processed foods is a much more economical way to eat. Below are the costs comparing a chicken and cheese tortilla to a vegetarian tortilla. As you can see, the more healthful vegetarian version costs about 40 percent less.

Nutrition facts: 690 calories, 56 grams protein, 44 grams fat, 17 grams carbohydrate (per serving)

8 small corn tortillas: $1.29

1 pound Kraft shredded cheddar cheese: $3.29

1 pound chicken breast: $3.48

1 (4-ounce) jar salsa: $1.50

Total cost of chicken and cheese tortilla meal: $9.56 ($2.39 per serving)

VEGETARIAN TORTILLA (SERVES 4)

Nutrition facts: 485 calories, 12 grams protein, 7.6 grams fat, 93 grams carbohydrate (per serving)

8 small corn tortillas: $1.29

1 pound brown rice: $1.19

1 (15-ounce) can vegetarian refried beans: $0.69

1 (4-ounce) jar salsa: $1.50

½ head shredded lettuce: $0.99

Total cost of vegetarian tortilla: $5.66 ($1.42 per serving)

Dietary Fat

QUESTION: *Is it good to avoid using oils in cooking? And what about nuts?*

ANSWER: By avoiding the use of added oil and minimizing your use of nuts, you can greatly reduce the fat content of your diet. Although vegetable oils and nuts generally contain less saturated fatty acids compared with animal fats (with the exception of coconut and palm oil), when it comes to calories and possibly even hormone production, total fat is what matters—regardless of whether it's a "good" or "bad" fat. There are many ways to prepare foods without oil, such as using water or vegetable broth for stir-fries and substituting applesauce, banana, or soy yogurt for oil or butter in baked goods and desserts.[15,16]

QUESTION: *Aren't there essential oils that you need to get from fish? Can plant sources provide these essential oils?*

ANSWER: Two essential fatty acids cannot be synthesized in the body and must be included in the diet. Their names—*linolenic* and *linoleic* acid—will never show up on a food label and are not important to remember. What is important is that these basic fats are used to build specialized fats called omega-3 and omega-6 fatty acids.

Omega-3 and omega-6 fatty acids are important in the normal functioning of all tissues of the body. Deficiencies are responsible for a host of symptoms and disorders including abnormalities in the liver and kidneys, changes in the blood, reduced growth rates, decreased immune function, and skin changes including dryness and scaliness. Adequate intake of the essential fatty acids may protect against these health problems and may also reduce the risk of atherosclerosis, heart disease, stroke, and symptoms associated with ulcerative colitis, menstrual pain, and joint pain.

Alpha-linolenic acid, the primary omega-3 fatty acid, is found in many vegetables, beans, and fruits. More concentrated sources include flaxseeds, soybean products, walnuts, and wheat germ. Adding flaxseed oil to your salad or grinding flaxseeds for your breakfast cereal are simple ways to incorporate extra omega-3 fatty acids into your diet. Corn, safflower, sunflower, and cottonseed oils are generally low in omega-3 and high in omega-6.

Gamma-linolenic acid, a healthful omega-6 oil, can be found in more rare oils, including black currant, borage, evening primrose, and hempseed oils.

Some people eat fish and use fish oils to obtain their omega-3s. However, plant-derived omegas-3s have none of the potential contaminants that fish contain, nor do they have the fish odor that can be apparent in the perspiration of people using fish oil. They also tend to be lower in saturated fats. Between 15 and 30 percent of fish oil is saturated fat, which is about double that of plant oils. Fish make their omega-3 oils from linolenic acid in plankton, just as mammals—including humans—synthesize omega-3s from land plants.[17,18]

Eggs

QUESTION: *Is there evidence linking the consumption of eggs to cancer risk?*

ANSWER: While egg consumption has not been studied as thoroughly as the consumption of meat and dairy products in relation to cancer risk, there is still enough evidence to encourage dietary alternatives to both egg whites and egg yolks. About 70 percent of the calories in eggs are from fat—a big portion of which is saturated fat. They are also loaded with cholesterol—about 213 milligrams for an average-sized egg. Eggs have no dietary fiber and are devoid of cancer-fighting antioxidants.

The most convincing evidence points to egg consumption as increasing risk for colorectal cancer and bladder cancer. The World Health Organization analyzed data from thirty-four countries and determined that egg consumption was significantly correlated with mortality from colon and rectal cancers in both men and women.[19] A study done in Argentina found that people who consumed approximately one and a half eggs per week had nearly five times more colorectal cancer risk than individuals consuming fewer than eleven eggs per year.[20] Moderate egg consumption also tripled the risk of developing bladder cancer, as determined by a study of 130 newly diagnosed bladder cancer patients published in the journal *International Urology and Nephrology*.[21]

Eggs are often used in baked products because of their binding and leavening properties. But smart cooks have found good substitutes. See table 20 (page 67) for tips on replacing eggs in recipes.

Food Safety

QUESTION: *How do you ensure proper food safety when cooking for someone undergoing chemotherapy?*

ANSWER: A clean and safe food supply is important for everyone, but is essential for people with compromised immune systems. Older persons and individuals undergoing cancer treatment are especially at risk from bacteria, viruses, or other foreign substances that can turn up in food. To keep your meals safe and clean, follow these simple practices:

- Wash your hands with soap and hot water before and after preparing food and before eating.
- Avoid preparing or eating all types of meat, eggs, and dairy products, as these foods are commonly contaminated with bacteria. Poultry products are especially likely to be contaminated. Raw milk and home-prepared ice creams or mayonnaise, as well as cake and cookie batter made with eggs, may easily contain infectious bacteria.
- Keep cold foods cold (below 40 degrees F) and hot foods hot (above 165 degrees F).
- Wash fruits and vegetables thoroughly under running water before using them.
- Wash the tops of cans before opening them.
- During food preparation, if you need to taste the food you are making, use a different utensil from the one used for stirring or serving.
- Do not taste food that looks or smells strange.

General Nutrition

QUESTION: *If a completely plant-based diet isn't possible for me, is it okay if I eliminate red meat and cheese and eat a low-fat diet with egg whites, chicken, fish, and skim milk in addition to lots of fruits and vegetables?*

ANSWER: Eliminating red meat and cheese is a start. However, you'll want to go further and base your diet on whole grains, legumes, vegetables, and fruit. Your diet will be much richer in cancer-fighting vitamins, minerals, fiber, and phytochemicals. Chicken and fish contain fat—including significant amounts of saturated fat—as well as cholesterol and other harmful compounds, so the most health-promoting diets avoid them completely.

Skim milk and egg whites contain animal protein and cholesterol and no fiber, vitamin C, or healthful complex carbohydrate.

An easy way to shift to a completely plant-based diet is to do it 100 percent for three weeks. In the process, you will adjust to new flavors and tastes. As those twenty-one days fly by, see how you feel. You'll realize that you feel a lot better (and perhaps lighter!) and that you don't miss the high-fat foods.

Juices and Juicing

QUESTION: *How do fruit and vegetable juices compare to eating these foods whole?*

ANSWER: As a rule of thumb, it's important to shoot for consuming at least three servings of fruit and four servings of vegetables every day. Since juice is not as high in fiber as whole fruit or vegetables, it is always best to consume the whole food whenever possible. It has been shown that diets higher in fiber are not only beneficial for protecting against a number of cancers and chronic illnesses, they also help fill you up so that you don't "fill out." Maintaining a healthy weight helps reduce cancer risk.

For people who don't enjoy eating lots of fruits and vegetables, juicing can be a way to bring these nutritious foods into their routine. One-half cup (4 fluid ounces) of juice can be considered the equivalent of a single serving of fruits or vegetables. Juice made in a high-powered blender that retains the fiber in the food is best. Alternatively, use the fibrous end-product that juicers produce by adding it to salads, soups, stir-fries, or pasta sauces.

Lung Cancer

QUESTION: *Are there any dietary factors that can help reduce the risk of lung cancer?*

ANSWER: Of course, it is essential to avoid tobacco. However, diet may play a role, too. A study published in 2000 suggested that isothiocyanates and other natural chemicals in broccoli, bok choy, cabbage, and other cruciferous vegetables may reduce lung cancer risk.[22] Of 18,000 men studied, those with detectable isothiocyanates in their blood had a 36 percent lower chance of developing lung cancer compared to those with none.

Food sources of these compounds are far preferable to supplements. In fact, beta-carotene taken in doses higher than those which occur naturally in plant foods can actually increase cancer risk. The lesson is simple: vegetables and fruits should be a generous part of the diet.

Macrobiotic Diets

QUESTION: *Are macrobiotic diets helpful in cancer prevention and survival?*

ANSWER: The word "macrobiotic" means "long life" and refers to a health-ful lifestyle, diet, and other recommendations related to eating that are good for overall well-being and thus are also effective in cancer prevention and survival. Macrobiotic diet guidelines are largely drawn from the principles of traditional Chinese medicine and emphasize balance, with a particular focus on grains, vegetables, beans, and bean products. The diet generally excludes animal products, although some macrobiotic practitioners include fish. People following macrobiotic diets who wish to include higher-protein foods while avoiding fish can choose beans or tofu dishes.

Numerous epidemiological studies have shown that a low-fat, plant-based diet is effective for cancer prevention and survival. There have been a great many remarkable case reports of individuals whose bleak cancer prognoses were dramatically improved though macrobiotics.[23]

Organic Food

QUESTION: *How important is it to choose organic foods?*

ANSWER: Buying organic produce is a good idea. It helps you avoid toxic chemicals and improve the nutritional value of the foods you eat. Table 18 (page 64) lists twenty-four fruits and vegetables with the highest and low-est levels of pesticide residue. Organically grown plant foods are not only more flavorful than conventionally grown crops, they are more nutritious and richer in cancer-fighting antioxidants and other phytochemicals.

Depending on where you live, you may find organic produce at your regular grocery store. You can also look for affordable organic food at a farmers' market in your area or join a community supported agriculture (CSA) group to receive local seasonal harvests. Not all organic farms are certified organic, because certification can be cost-prohibitive for smaller farmers. However, by buying local produce you can learn personally from farmers about their farming practices and ensure that you are getting safe fresh produce.

"Organic" meat is another story. Buying organic meat does not nec-essarily mean that you are eliminating the health risks associated with the consumption of animal products. For instance, heterocyclic amines (HCAs), a family of mutagenic compounds, are produced during the process of cooking chicken, beef, pork, and fish. Meat that is cooked under normal grilling temperatures commonly contains significant quanti-ties of these carcinogens. The longer and hotter the meat is cooked, the more these compounds form. There is also significant evidence that con-suming dairy products, conventional or organic, may increase blood levels of IGF-1, a hormone in the body that has been associated with increased cancer risk. And both meat and dairy, regardless of whether or not they are organic, can provide considerable amounts of saturated fat and cholesterol.

Choosing a plant-based diet that is also low in pollutants and pesticide residues will enable you to control some of the major factors that have been linked to the risk of cancer and other degenerative diseases.[24,25]

Protein

QUESTION: *How do you get enough protein on a vegan diet?*

ANSWER: That is very easy. Here's what you need to know: Protein is used for the building, maintenance, and repair of tissues in the body. Amino acids, the building blocks of protein, are synthesized by the body or ingested from food. There are nine essential amino acids that cannot be produced by the body and must be obtained from the diet. A variety of grains, legumes, and vegetables easily provides all of the essential amino acids our bodies require. It was once thought that various plant foods had to be eaten in specific combinations to get their full protein value. We now know that intentional food combining is not necessary. When the diet contains a variety of grains, legumes, and vegetables, protein needs are easily met.

On average, North Americans consume about double the amount of protein they actually need. Because North Americans tend to rely on animal products, they get a significant amount of saturated fat and cholesterol along with their protein. The recommended daily intake of protein for the average, sedentary adult is only about one-third of a gram (0.36 gram to be exact) of protein per pound of body weight. For those using metric weights, this is 0.8 gram per kilogram of body weight.

To calculate your recommended amount, simply multiply your weight (in pounds) by 0.36. This value has a large margin of safety, and the body's true need is actually lower for most people. Protein needs are somewhat higher for women who are pregnant or breastfeeding compared to other women. Needs are also higher for very active persons. As these groups require additional calories, increased protein needs can easily be met simply through larger intake of food. Extra servings of legumes, tofu, meat alternatives, or other plant-based sources of concentrated protein can easily meet needs that go beyond the recommendation for sedentary adults.

Raw Food Diets

QUESTION: *What about raw food vegan diets? Are they even better than vegan diets that include cooked foods?*

ANSWER: Few studies have evaluated the health benefits of raw food diets. However, a low-fat diet that is rich in raw or cooked vegetables, fruits, and other plant-based foods is loaded with antioxidants and other cancer-fighting nutrients. There are significant advantages to having vegetables and fruits in their raw form, because cooking sometimes causes the loss of some nutrients that are powerful antioxidants and help protect us from developing cancer.

Salt

QUESTION: *Does salt increase cancer risk? How do table salt, sea salt, and kosher salt differ?*

ANSWER: Studies in Asia suggest that consuming foods preserved by salting and pickling is associated with increased risk for stomach cancer.[26] Also, when salt intake exceeds about 2 grams per day the risk of hypertension increases, as does the loss of calcium through the kidneys. However, using modest amounts of salt in cooking or for flavoring foods does not appear to increase the risk of health problems.

Table salt, sea salt, and kosher salt all have the same sodium content, but they differ in taste and texture. Sea salt comes from evaporated seawater, whereas table salt and kosher salt come from rock salt from inland deposits. Sea salt can be either fine or coarse and often has a flavor that is slightly different from table or kosher salt because of the additional minerals it contains. Table salt is fine in texture and often has added iodine, which is necessary for proper thyroid function. Other additives in table salt may include the following: sodium hexacyanoferrate (II), tricalcium phosphate, calcium carbonate, magnesium carbonate, fatty acid salts, acid salts, magnesium oxide, silicon dioxide, calcium silicate, sodium aluminosilicate, and alumino-calcium silicate. Kosher salt is coarse-grained and usually has no additives.

Soy

QUESTION: *Do the phytoestrogens in soy foods prevent cancer? Are they helpful or risky for cancer survivors? What about the estrogens in soy for men and boys?*

ANSWER: Soy products, such as miso soup, tofu, and tempeh, contain very weak plant estrogens called *phytoestrogens*, which block the body's natural estrogen from attaching to cells.[27] (The prefix "phyto" simply means "plant.") Normally, estrogens hook onto tiny receptor proteins on your cells that allow them to influence the cell's chemistry.

Think of it this way: An estrogen molecule is like a jumbo jet that attaches to the Jetway of an airport. It discharges passengers into the terminal, which is suddenly a busy, noisy place. Phytoestrogens, being weak estrogens, are like small, private planes with few passengers and no cargo, yet they still occupy the Jetway after landing. When phytoestrogens occupy the cellular receptors, normal estrogens cannot. So, while plant estrogens do not eliminate all of estrogen's effects, they do minimize them, apparently reducing breast cancer risk and menstrual symptoms.[28,29]

Like all foods, soy products have advantages and disadvantages. Soybeans are rich in essential omega-3 fatty acids, but they tend to be higher in fat compared to other beans. Many soy products derive roughly half their calories from fat, while black beans, pinto beans, or other varieties are only about 4 percent fat. Also, soy extracts, such as genistein, may not have the same beneficial effects as products made with the whole bean.

In Asia, where tofu, soymilk, and other soy products are commonly consumed, not only is the population healthier overall, but cancer and heart disease are much rarer than in North America and Europe and longevity is greater. However, these populations differ in other ways, aside from their use of soy products. Asians eat much less meat and dairy products and generally exercise more compared to Americans; they also smoke more cigarettes and eat more salt. It has therefore been difficult for researchers to tease out the effects of soy itself.

Also, it is possible that soy products that go through more processing, such as veggie burgers, veggie hot dogs, and particularly isolated soy protein products, are not as beneficial as soy products with less processing, such as whole soybeans, tofu, and tempeh, which are traditionally consumed in Asia. Replacing processed soy products with more traditional, less processed ones, or with other whole beans and lentils, may provide you with a more health-promoting diet.

In human research studies, soy products have been shown to lower blood cholesterol levels, in part due to their rich content of soluble fiber, and their isoflavones also play a role in bone formation. Soy products have been shown to reduce estrogen activity, at least in premenopausal women, which, over the long run, reduces cancer risk. The evidence is not as definitive for postmenopausal women.

Research findings are not clear on whether soy products are safe for women who have had breast cancer. Some researchers believe that two servings per day of soy products, such as soymilk, tofu, or tempeh, are fine for these women, while others discourage soy consumption completely. It is also not yet clear whether the effects of soy products differ for women with estrogen receptor-positive breast cancer compared to those with estrogen receptor-negative cancers.

For men and boys, the phytoestrogens in soy do not appear to have any adverse effect on hormone levels and have not been shown to affect sexual development or fertility.[30] Research studies show that men consuming soy have less prostate cancer and better prostate cancer survival.

However, it's also important to remember that a vegan diet of beans, vegetables, grains, and fruits does not have to include soy products to be nutritionally complete. Soy products make convenient alternatives for meat and other health-damaging foods that people, quite rightly, are looking to avoid. However, the benefits of complete protein and soluble fiber can easily be found in an array of plant foods.

Sugar

QUESTION: *How important is it to steer clear of sugar? I've heard that sugar feeds cancer cells.*

ANSWER: Simple sugars (syrup, honey, white sugar, brown sugar, soda) provide calories but no nutritional benefit when it comes to cancer prevention and survival. It is easy to overdo it with simple sugars because they are not filling. They can promote weight gain, which increases the risk for certain cancer types. In addition, there's some evidence that the elevated insulin levels resulting from the consumption of simple sugars may increase cancer risk and potentially impair survival. For these reasons, it's important to limit your intake of simple sugars and choose more wholesome sweet foods, such as fruits, which have cancer-fighting nutrients and fiber.[31,32]

Supplements

QUESTION: *Do you recommend taking the popular "green food" supplements that are on the market now? Will they help prevent cancer?*

ANSWER: Vegetable-based supplements are increasing in popularity and often come with a variety of health claims. Whether or not they have benefit, it is important to consider that no single supplement can replicate all the healthful components found in a variety of whole plant foods, including those that ward off cancer. Vegetables, fruits, whole grains, and legumes are packed with healthful substances *beyond* vitamins, such as fiber, minerals, and cancer-protective phytochemicals. Increasing your fruits and vegetables can be almost as simple as popping a pill and is far more beneficial. Try these simple ideas to get your seven (or more) servings a day:

- Add vitamin-rich veggies, such as bell peppers, broccoli, carrots, spinach, and tomatoes to salads.
- Add puréed cooked pumpkin or winter squash to soups and stews as a thickener.
- Take a bowl of fruit to work each week (apples, bananas, oranges, pears) and snack on them when hunger calls.
- Pack raisins and other dried fruits in your purse, briefcase, or backpack to keep you fueled with wholesome foods.

One supplement that is important, however, is vitamin B_{12}, which is needed for healthy blood and nerves. It is found in any common multiple vitamin and in simple B_{12} supplements. It is also found in fortified cereals, fortified soymilks, and some brands of nutritional yeast.

Tea

QUESTION: *Is tea beneficial for cancer prevention?*

ANSWER: Perhaps. A recent study followed 69,000 Chinese women ages forty to seventy and found that the more green tea consumed, the lower the risk of developing colorectal cancer.[33] The same effect has not been found for oral cancer, gastric cancer, and perhaps for cancer in general. However, it appears that there is a lower mortality rate among consumers of regular green tea. Some have suggested that the health benefits of green tea stem from the antioxidant properties of polyphenolic compounds, or catechins, which are especially high in green tea due to its unique preparation. Catechins can be found in many different types of teas, not just green tea; however, the concentrations are inconsistent and variable.

Catechins make up 30 percent of the weight of the dried green tea leaves. It is known that antioxidant levels increase in the blood after green tea consumption, but the implications of this for health are unclear. More research is needed to understand green tea and its antioxidant activity in the human body. However, some clinical trials investigating green tea consumption by cancer patients found potential benefits that may prove promising.[34,35]

Treatment

QUESTION: *Is a vegan diet recommended for patients who have just been diagnosed with cancer and are not undergoing therapy yet but are about to have surgery?*

ANSWER: The information in this book is intended for individuals interested in prevention and those who are done with treatment. While a vegan diet can be healthful and beneficial at all stages of life, anyone undergoing medical treatment should talk with his or her doctor about any major dietary changes.

Weight Control

QUESTION: *I'm underweight and having trouble keeping weight on. What are some nutritious plant-based snacks that will prevent me from losing weight?*

ANSWER: Dried beans and peas, nuts, and seeds are examples of foods can help. They supply both calories and protein, among other nutrients. Shakes can be made with rice milk, almond milk, soymilk, tofu, and nondairy frozen desserts and can be flavored with frozen or fresh fruit and vanilla or other extracts to make tasty, calorie-rich treats. Also, dried fruit is rich in calories and nutrients but low in fat, and many varieties of trail mix are easily available and great for high-energy snacking.

QUESTION: *For an overweight breast cancer survivor, is it important to just focus on eating healthfully, or is weight loss important also?*

ANSWER: You will want to focus on both. Evidence suggests you can improve your chances of surviving breast cancer and reduce recurrence by achieving a healthy weight. The best way to lose weight is to choose health-promoting, low-fat meals built around legumes, grains, vegetables, and fruit, and incorporate more physical activity into your lifestyle. Of course, it's important to check with your doctor first to get the green light on the type and level of exercise you'd like to do. Once you get the go-ahead, make a commitment to regular exercise. You'll feel better for it!

Nutrition Basics

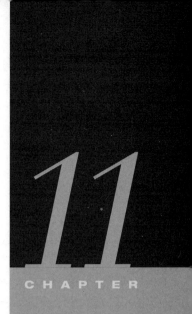

L et us define the basic terms nutrition experts use in planning health-promoting diets. What do we mean when we talk about carbohydrate, protein, and fat? What are they for, and how much (or how little) of each should we be getting each day?

Good nutrition means getting these nutrients, along with fiber, vitamins, and minerals, not only in the right amounts, but also in the right form. This chapter will help you understand the basics of the macronutrients (carbohydrate, protein, and fat) and fiber—why we need them, and what the most healthful choices are.

Carbohydrate

Carbohydrate is the main source of energy in a health-supporting diet. It is the primary fuel source for the brain and muscles and helps maintain nervous system function. Normally, your body stores a bit of carbohydrate in your muscles and liver as *glycogen*, which acts as a reserve energy source. Liver glycogen maintains blood glucose levels, but it is soon depleted if no carbohydrate is consumed. When that happens, your body can make carbohydrate from amino acids that are drawn from your muscles, but that means that your muscle mass will dwindle.

There are two types of carbohydrate: simple and complex. The term *simple carbohydrate* refers to sugars found in fruits or in concentrated forms, such as table sugar.

Complex carbohydrate, or starch, is composed of many sugar molecules joined together. The following are some common foods that are rich in complex carbohydrate:

- beans
- potatoes
- vegetables
- whole grains

It is remarkably easy to get enough protein. A variety of grains, legumes, and vegetables can provide all of the essential amino acids our bodies require.

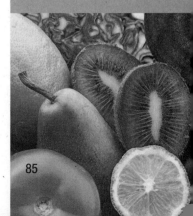

Generally speaking, you will want to favor foods rich in complex carbohydrate. For most people, 55–75 percent of daily calories should come from carbohydrate.

Fiber

Fiber is only found in plant foods. This is why vegetarians, particularly vegans, often have a high fiber intake. Fiber provides us with many benefits, including reduced cancer risk, as we saw in chapter 2. Fiber intake is one of the reasons vegetarians have significantly lower rates of cancer, heart disease, and diabetes and are usually slimmer than other people. Fiber helps you to fill up so that you don't "fill out."

The two types of fiber are *insoluble* and *soluble*. It is important to have both insoluble and soluble fiber in your diet. Most foods contain a mixture of both fibers, and the two types are not usually differentiated on food labels.

Insoluble fiber does not readily dissolve in water. It increases fecal bulk and decreases intestinal transit time. All plants, especially vegetables, wheat, wheat bran, rye, and rice, are rich in insoluble fiber.

Soluble fiber dissolves or swells when it is put into water and is readily metabolized by intestinal bacteria. It has been shown to help lower cholesterol levels and slow down gastric emptying time (thus keeping you full longer). Beans, fruits, and oats are especially good sources of soluble fiber. Other examples of soluble fiber include guar gum and locust bean gum—these are commonly used as thickeners and found in salad dressings and jams.

Most health authorities recommended fiber intake in the range of 25–35 grams per day as a minimal goal, and, optimally, your goal should be about 40 grams. The average American eats 14–15 grams a day, and vegetarians get two to three times that amount. Increase your fiber intake slowly, and increase water intake as well. Here is the fiber content of some common foods:

- beans: about 7 grams per ½-cup serving
- fruits: about 3 grams per average fruit
- vegetables: about 4 grams per 1-cup serving

Protein

Protein is needed to build and repair muscles, bone, skin, and blood; regulate hormones and enzymes; and help fight infection and heal wounds. It is also an integral part of genes and chromosomes.

The building blocks of protein are called *amino acids*. The body can synthesize some amino acids; others must be ingested from food. Of the twenty or so different amino acids in the food we eat, our bodies can make eleven. The nine remaining amino acids are called *essential amino acids*—that is, the body cannot produce them, and they must be obtained from the diet.

TABLE 22 Higher-protein plant foods

FOOD	SERVING SIZE	CALORIES	PROTEIN (GRAMS)	FAT (GRAMS)
All-Bran cereal	1 cup	213	8.0	1.5
black beans, cooked	1 cup	227	15.2	0.9
chickpeas, cooked	1 cup	285	11.9	2.7
Grape-Nuts cereal	1 cup	416	12.4	0.4
kidney beans, cooked	1 cup	225	15.4	0.9
lentils, cooked	1 cup	231	17.9	0.7
pinto beans, cooked	1 cup	235	14.0	0.9
soymilk	1 cup	140	10.0	4.0
split peas, cooked	1 cup	231	16.4	0.8
tempeh burger	1 burger	110	12.5	3.2
textured vegetable protein, rehydrated	1 cup	120	22.0	0.2
tofu (firm)	1 cup	366	39.8	22.0
vegetarian baked beans	1 cup	235	12.2	1.1

It is remarkably easy to get enough protein. A variety of grains, legumes, and vegetables can provide all of the essential amino acids our bodies require. It was once thought that to get adequate protein various plant foods had to be consumed together, a practice known as protein combining or protein complementing. However, researchers have found that intentional combining is not necessary. As long as the diet contains a variety of grains, legumes, and vegetables, protein needs are easily met.

Approximately 10–15 percent of daily calories should come from protein. Protein needs depend on body weight, and requirements increase with activity level and body stress (such as tissue repair or medical treatments). All foods except pure fats, sugars, and alcohol contain protein. The recommended dietary allowance (RDA) for protein for the average sedentary adult is only 0.8 grams per kilogram of body weight, with protein needs increasing only slightly with more activity. To find out your average individual need, simply perform the following calculation: body weight (in pounds) x 0.36 = recommended protein intake (in grams).

Here is an example: A person who weighs 150 pounds needs 54 grams of protein per day. What does 54 grams of protein look like on a full day's menu?

Breakfast: 1 bowl of bran cereal with raisins and 1 cup of soymilk   12 grams

Lunch: 1 veggie burger on a whole wheat bun   20 grams

Dinner: 1 cup of pasta with 1 cup of assorted vegetables and beans   22 grams

Protein Total for the Day   54 grams

The most protein-rich plant foods are listed in table 22. Legumes (beans, peas, and lentils) are especially rich in many healthful nutrients and supply a substantial amount of protein. Most varieties of legumes are about 25 percent protein and yield approximately 15 grams of protein per cup. But don't think that beans have a patent on protein. Wheat noodles contain substantial amounts; some varieties have about 10 grams of protein in every 2 ounces of dried pasta, and that's before you figure in any toppings.

Fat

Fat is the most concentrated source of calories. Any sort of fat—chicken fat, fish fat, beef fat, or vegetable oil—has 9 calories per gram, more than twice the calorie content of carbohydrate or protein. Most health authorities recommend that fat intake not exceed 30 percent of our calories. This means that a person consuming 2,000 calories per day should have less than 60 grams of fat per day.

However, research has shown that the lower your fat intake, the better your chances of warding off heart disease and cancer and keeping your waistline slim. A healthier goal is to limit fat to about 25–35 grams per day.

Fats are made up of a combination of *fatty acids*, which can be *monounsaturated*, *polyunsaturated*, or *saturated*. All fats contain some of each of these three, but health authorities have long recommended minimizing saturated fats because of their tendency to raise cholesterol levels. Animal products are generally very high in saturated fatty acids, whereas vegetable oils are generally much lower in this type of fat. There are a few exceptions: coconut oil, palm oil, and palm kernel oil are quite high in saturated fat.

Fat is necessary for the structure and maintenance of cells and hormones, healthy skin and hair, and the metabolism of fat-soluble vitamins (A, D, E, and K). As long as we consume enough calories, we can synthesize fat from surplus protein and carbohydrates. However, there are two *essential fatty acids* that we need to obtain from our diet. They are *alpha-linolenic acid* (an omega-3 fatty acid) and *linoleic acid* (an omega-6 fatty acid). Both are important in the normal functioning of all tissues of the body. Deficiencies are responsible for a host of symptoms and disorders, including abnormalities in the liver and kidney, changes in the blood, reduced growth rates, decreased immune function, and skin changes, such as dryness and scaliness. Adequate intake of the essential fatty acids results in numerous health benefits, including reduced incidence of heart disease and stroke and relief from the symptoms associated with ulcerative colitis, menstrual pain, and joint pain.

Most people consume too many omega-6 fatty acids and too few omega-3 fatty acids. It's important to maintain a balance of these two. Omega-6 fatty acids are present in higher concentrations in many foods, whereas omega-3 fatty acids are not as widespread. Beans, vegetables, fruits, and whole grains do contain omega-3 fatty acids, but the most concentrated plant sources include canola oil, flaxseeds, wheat germ, soybeans, and walnuts.

Recipes

12

CHAPTER

N
ow that you understand the science behind following a plant-based diet, it's time to head into the kitchen. The recipes in this chapter have been written and modified to appeal to both novice and experienced chefs. When there are ingredients that may be new to you, the recipe introduction explains what those ingredients are and why they're being used in that particular recipe.

In compiling the recipes, we've taken into account busy lifestyles and convenience. We encourage you to experiment with a variety of plant foods and to modify ingredients based on your personal preferences. For example, if you would rather use beans or tofu instead of seitan (a chewy meat alternative made from wheat) in any recipe that calls for it, please feel free to. When you are preparing the recipes, keep in mind that whole, unprocessed foods are the richest in health-promoting nutrients. We do not expect you to love every single recipe, but we do hope that you'll find many to include in your daily menus.

When reviewing the nutritional analysis for each of the recipes, remember that The Cancer Project recommends a low-fat diet that limits fat to 10–20 percent of calories. Some of the recipes have more than 20 percent of calories from fat, and many have less than 5 percent. Eaten over a day or week's time, all of the recipes can be included in a health-promoting plan, as they are generally low in total fat and calories. Enjoy experimenting with these healthful new foods!

designates recipes that take less than 30 minutes to prepare

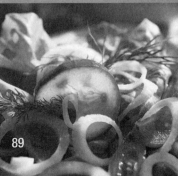

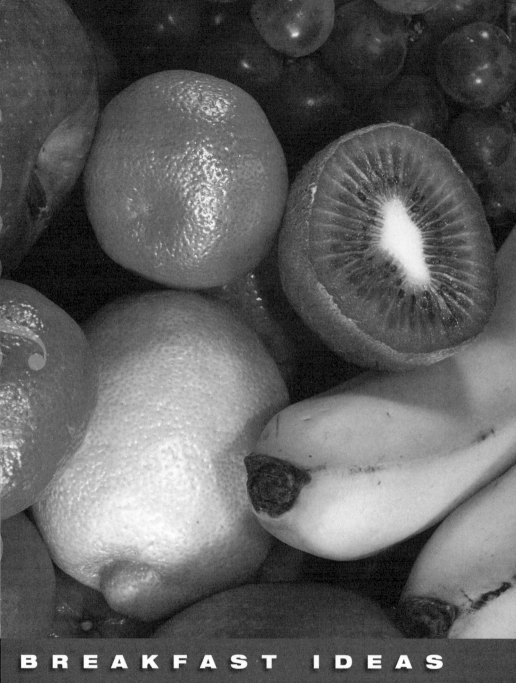

Breakfast

BREAKFAST IDEAS

Banana-Oat Pancakes

These satisfying pancakes contain generous amounts of heart-healthful oats. They are delicious when served with orange slices or other fresh fruit, or a bit of real maple syrup. You can purchase oat flour at natural food stores and in some supermarkets, or you can make your own by grinding rolled oats in a food processor or blender.

1 cup oat flour

¼ cup whole wheat pastry flour

½ teaspoon baking soda

⅛ teaspoon salt

1 cup fortified soymilk or other nondairy milk

1 ripe banana, mashed

¼ cup chopped walnuts (optional)

1 tablespoon maple syrup

1½ teaspoons apple cider vinegar

1. Combine the oat flour, pastry flour, baking soda, and salt in a small bowl and stir to mix.

2. Combine the soymilk, banana, optional walnuts, maple syrup, and vinegar in a medium bowl and mix thoroughly.

3. To make the batter, add the flour mixture to the soymilk mixture and stir just until combined.

4. Heat a large nonstick skillet. Pour small amounts of the batter onto the heated skillet and cook until the tops bubble and the edges are dry. Turn the pancakes over and cook the other side for about 1 minute, until golden brown. Serve immediately.

5. Stored in a covered container in the refrigerator, leftover Banana-Oat Pancakes will keep for up to 2 days.

PER SERVING: 78 calories; 1.1 g fat; 0.2 g saturated fat; 13.1% calories from fat; 0 mg cholesterol; 3 g protein; 14.8 g carbohydrate; 3.5 g sugar; 2 g fiber; 107 mg sodium; 38 mg calcium; 0.8 mg iron; 1.1 mg vitamin C; 3 mcg beta-carotene; 0.4 mg vitamin E

Breakfast Home Fries

T hese low-fat home-fried potatoes make a delicious breakfast or side dish any time of day. Serve them with applesauce or alongside Black Bean Chili (page 121) and Mango Salsa (page 111).

3 russet potatoes, scrubbed

1 onion, thinly sliced

4 teaspoons soy sauce

½ teaspoon paprika or chili powder

¼ teaspoon ground black pepper

5 or 6 cherry tomatoes, cut into quarters (optional)

2 green onions, thinly sliced (optional)

1. Cut the potatoes into ½-inch cubes and steam them for about 10 minutes, or until just tender. Remove from the heat and set aside.

2. Heat ¼ cup of water in a large nonstick skillet and add the onion. Cook, stirring frequently, until the water has evaporated and the onion begins to stick to the pan. Scrape the pan as you add another ¼ cup of water, and continue cooking until the onion once again begins to stick. Repeat this process until the onion is very brown and sweet. This will take about 15 minutes.

3. Add the potatoes to the skillet with the onion and sprinkle with the soy sauce, paprika, and pepper. Cook, turning the mixture gently with a spatula, until the potatoes are golden brown. If desired, garnish with the tomatoes and green onions.

4. Stored in a covered container in the refrigerator, leftover Breakfast Home Fries will keep for up to 3 days.

PER SERVING: 128 calories; 0.2 g fat; 0.1 g saturated fat; 1.7% calories from fat; 0 mg cholesterol; 3.1 g protein; 29.9 g carbohydrate; 2.7 g sugar; 4.1 g fiber; 309 mg sodium; 39 mg calcium; 2.7 mg iron; 19.5 mg vitamin C; 89 mcg beta-carotene; 0.2 mg vitamin E

Breakfast Scramble

This is a low-fat, cholesterol-free way to enjoy scrambled "eggs." Using tofu instead of eggs provides healthful plant protein. Turmeric gives the scramble an appealing golden color.

1 pound low-fat tofu

1 teaspoon dried parsley flakes, lightly crumbled

½ teaspoon ground turmeric

¼ teaspoon salt

¼ teaspoon ground black pepper

2 tablespoons vegetable broth

½ medium onion, chopped

2 garlic cloves, minced

1 green bell pepper, diced

1 red bell pepper, diced

1 medium zucchini, diced

1. Press the block of tofu between two plates to remove excess liquid. Place a few paper towels between the tofu and the bottom plate, and put a can of vegetables or a similar weight on the top plate. Replace the paper towels with fresh ones as they become saturated. Press the tofu for at least 30 minutes or up to 2 hours; the longer you press it, the firmer it will become.

2. Combine the parsley, turmeric, salt, and pepper in a small dish. Heat the vegetable broth in a medium skillet. Add the onion and garlic and cook and stir until they are tender. Add the bell peppers and zucchini and cook and stir until they are soft.

3. Crumble the tofu into the skillet and sprinkle with the parsley mixture. Cook and stir over medium heat until hot throughout.

4. Stored in a covered container in the refrigerator, leftover Breakfast Scramble will keep for up to 2 days.

PER SERVING: 86 calories; 3.5 g fat; 0.5 g saturated fat; 40.8% calories from fat; 0 mg cholesterol; 6.9 g protein; 8.7 g carbohydrate; 3.2 g sugar; 3.3 g fiber; 122 mg sodium; 51 mg calcium; 2.4 mg iron; 49.4 mg vitamin C; 608 mcg beta-carotene; 0.6 mg vitamin E

Fruited Breakfast Quinoa

Quinoa is technically a seed, but it is treated like a grain in cooking and was a highly nutritious staple in the diet of the ancient Incas. It has a delicious flavor and a light, fluffy texture. It is important to rinse quinoa thoroughly prior to cooking to remove the bitter resinlike coating called saponin.

1½ cups vanilla rice milk

½ cup quinoa, rinsed and drained

1 cup chopped fresh or canned apricots

2 tablespoons raisins

¼ teaspoon vanilla extract

1. Combine the rice milk and quinoa in a medium saucepan. Bring to a gentle simmer. Cover and cook for about 15 minutes, until the quinoa is tender.

2. Stir in the apricots, raisins, and vanilla extract. Cover and cook for 2 minutes longer. Serve warm or chilled.

3. Stored in a covered container in the refrigerator, leftover Fruited Breakfast Quinoa will keep for up to 3 days.

PER SERVING: 106 calories; 1.4 g fat; 0.1 g saturated fat; 12.3% calories from fat; 0 mg cholesterol; 2.4 g protein; 21.4 g carbohydrate; 8.3 g sugar; 1.5 g fiber; 26 mg sodium; 90 mg calcium; 1.5 mg iron; 3.1 mg vitamin C; 302 mcg beta-carotene; 0.9 mg vitamin E

How to Rinse Quinoa

To thoroughly rinse quinoa, cover it with water in a mixing bowl and rub it between the palms of your hands. Pour off the cloudy liquid through a strainer. Repeat the process two or three more times, or until the rinse water remains clear.

Tofu French Toast

 ofu works just like eggs when it comes to french toast, without the cholesterol and saturated fat that eggs would normally contribute.

8 ounces low-fat silken tofu

1 ripe banana

½ cup water

1 teaspoon light molasses or maple syrup

½ teaspoon ground cinnamon

6 slices whole wheat bread

1. Combine the tofu, banana, water, molasses, and cinnamon in a blender and process until smooth. Pour into a shallow dish.

2. Place a nonstick skillet over medium heat. Dip each slice of bread into the banana mixture and brown it on both sides in the skillet. You will need to brown the bread in several batches depending on the size of your skillet.

3. Stored in a covered container in the refrigerator, leftover Tofu French Toast will keep for up to 2 days.

PER SERVING: 123 calories; 2.9 g fat; 0.5 g saturated fat; 21.4% calories from fat; 0 mg cholesterol; 6.1 g protein; 20.4 g carbohydrate; 6.1 g sugar; 3.6 g fiber; 151 mg sodium; 46 mg calcium; 2.1 mg iron; 2.1 mg vitamin C; 7 mcg beta-carotene; 0.2 mg vitamin E

Applesauce Muffins

hese delicious, low-fat muffins take just thirty minutes to assemble and bake. Plus, they don't use eggs or butter, which eliminates a great deal of unhealthful fat and all of the cholesterol.

2½ cups whole wheat pastry flour

¼ cup sugar

1 teaspoon ground cinnamon

½ teaspoon baking soda

¼ teaspoon ground nutmeg

¼ teaspoon salt

1 cup unsweetened applesauce

½ cup fortified soymilk or other nondairy milk

1 tablespoon vegetable oil

1 tablespoon light molasses

1 tablespoon apple cider vinegar

½ cup raisins

1. Preheat the oven to 375 degrees F. Lightly mist 10 muffin cups with vegetable oil spray.

2. Combine the flour, sugar, cinnamon, baking soda, nutmeg, and salt in a medium bowl and mix thoroughly.

3. Combine the applesauce, soymilk, oil, molasses, and vinegar in a large bowl and mix thoroughly. Add the flour mixture and stir until just combined. Stir in the raisins.

4. Spoon the batter into the prepared muffin cups, filling them about three-quarters full. Bake for 15 to 20 minutes, or until a toothpick inserted into the center of a muffin comes out clean.

5. Stored in a covered container in the refrigerator, Applesauce Muffins will keep for up to 3 days. If longer storage is needed, freeze the cooled muffins in heavy-duty zipper-lock bags for up to 1 month. Defrost at room temperature or in a microwave.

Variation: Add ¼ cup of chopped walnuts to the batter and/or replace the raisins with ½ cup of dried cranberries.

PER SERVING: 178 calories; 2.2 g fat; 0.3 g saturated fat; 11.1% calories from fat; 0 mg cholesterol; 4.8 g protein; 37.7 g carbohydrate; 12.5 g sugar; 4.5 g fiber; 134 mg sodium; 41 mg calcium; 1.7 mg iron; 0.6 mg vitamin C; 5 mcg beta-carotene; 0.6 mg vitamin E

Banana-Date Muffins

MAKES 10 MUFFINS (10 SERVINGS)

When your bananas develop brown speckles, they're ready for action! Freeze them for smoothies (see page 100), or use them to make these delicious banana muffins. With over 5 grams of fiber per muffin, these make a nutritious and filling snack.

2½ cups whole wheat pastry flour

½ teaspoon baking soda

¼ teaspoon salt

2 ripe bananas, mashed (about 1 cup)

1 cup fortified soymilk or other nondairy milk

½ cup sugar

1 tablespoon apple cider vinegar

1 teaspoon vanilla extract

½ cup chopped dates

1. Preheat the oven to 375 degrees F. Lightly mist 10 muffin cups with vegetable oil spray.
2. Combine the flour, baking soda, and salt in a small bowl.
3. Combine the bananas, soymilk, sugar, vinegar, and vanilla extract in a large bowl and mix thoroughly. Add the flour mixture and stir until just combined. Stir in the dates.
4. Spoon the batter into the prepared muffin cups, filling them about three-quarters full. Bake for about 25 minutes, or until a toothpick inserted into the center of a muffin comes out clean.
5. Stored in a covered container in the refrigerator, Banana-Date Muffins will keep for up to 3 days. If longer storage is needed, freeze the cooled muffins in heavy-duty zipper-lock bags for up to 1 month. Defrost at room temperature or in a microwave.

PER SERVING: 199 calories; 1.1 g fat; 0.2 g saturated fat; 4.9% calories from fat; 0 mg cholesterol; 5.4 g protein; 45.2 g carbohydrate; 18.8 g sugar; 5.3 g fiber; 142 mg sodium; 53 mg calcium; 1.8 mg iron; 2.2 mg vitamin C; 8 mcg beta-carotene; 0.6 mg vitamin E

Sweet Potato Muffins

U se leftover sweet potatoes from last night's dinner to make these luscious muffins. You can use any variety of sweet potato; each will give a slightly different result, all of them nutritious and delicious.

3 cups whole wheat pastry flour

½ cup sugar

1 tablespoon baking powder

1 teaspoon ground cinnamon

½ teaspoon baking soda

½ teaspoon salt

1 cup cooked and mashed sweet potato

1 cup fortified soymilk or other nondairy milk

1 tablespoon apple cider vinegar

1 cup golden raisins

1. Preheat the oven to 375 degrees F. Lightly mist 12 muffin cups with vegetable oil spray.

2. Combine the flour, sugar, baking powder, cinnamon, baking soda, and salt in a small bowl and mix thoroughly.

3. Stir together the sweet potatoes, soymilk, and vinegar in a large bowl. Add the flour mixture and raisins and mix until just combined. The batter should be moist. Add a bit more nondairy milk or water if the batter seems stiff.

4. Spoon the batter into the prepared muffin cups, filling them almost to the top. Bake for about 25 minutes, or until the tops of the muffins bounce back when lightly touched and a toothpick inserted into the center of a muffin comes out clean.

5. Stored in a covered container in the refrigerator, Sweet Potato Muffins will keep for up to 3 days. If longer storage is needed, freeze the cooled muffins in heavy-duty zipper-lock bags for up to 1 month. Defrost at room temperature or in a microwave.

PER SERVING: 198 calories; 1 g fat; 0.2 g saturated fat; 4.5% calories from fat; 0 mg cholesterol; 5.6 g protein; 45.1 g carbohydrate; 17.2 g sugar; 5.1 g fiber; 297 mg sodium; 125 mg calcium; 2.1 mg iron; 4.1 mg vitamin C; 2188 mcg beta-carotene; 0.7 mg vitamin E

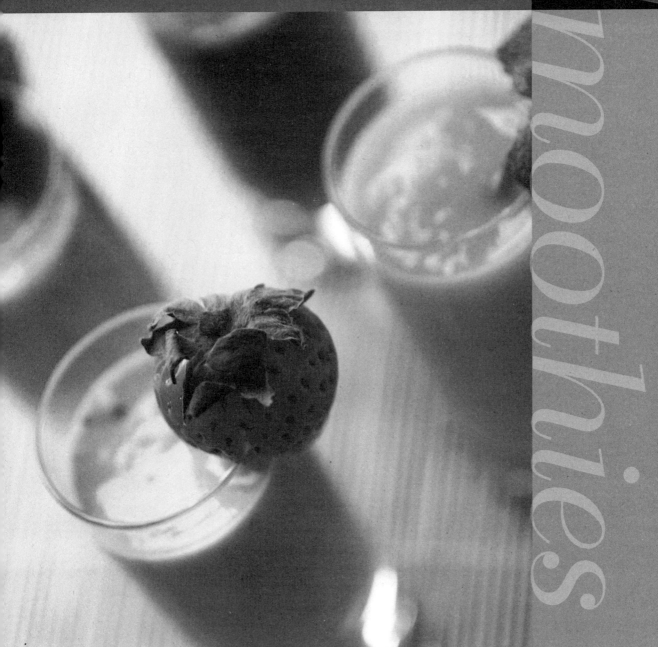

Blueberry Smoothie

Smoothies are a delicious way to add healthful fruits to your diet. Frozen berries can be purchased at most supermarkets and natural food stores. To freeze your own, loosely pack clean, dry berries in a heavy-duty zipper-lock plastic bag or storage container. For a thick smoothie that can be eaten with a spoon, use the minimum amount of soymilk necessary for blending; if you prefer a thinner smoothie, simply add a bit more.

1½ cups frozen blueberries

1 cup frozen banana chunks (see sidebar)

½ to 1 cup fortified soymilk or other nondairy milk

1 tablespoon apple juice concentrate

1. Combine all of the ingredients in a blender and process until smooth. Stop the blender occasionally to scrape down the sides of the container and push any unblended fruit into the blades with a rubber spatula.

2. Blueberry Smoothie is best served immediately. Leftovers may be stored in the refrigerator for up to 1 day or frozen for up to 1 week. Blend the mixture again before serving.

PER SERVING: 213 calories; 1.9 g fat; 0.3 g saturated fat; 7.8% calories from fat; 0 mg cholesterol; 4.3 g protein; 50 g carbohydrate; 31.1 g sugar; 6.8 g fiber; 40 mg sodium; 91 mg calcium; 1.4 mg iron; 23.6 mg vitamin C; 75 mcg beta-carotene; 1.9 mg vitamin E

How to Freeze Bananas

Frozen fruit, especially frozen bananas, make it possible to create thick, low-fat smoothies. Start with bananas that have brown speckles, as they will be sweet and ripe. Peel them, break them into chunks, and arrange the pieces on a baking sheet or tray to freeze. Once frozen, pack them loosely into heavy-duty zipper-lock plastic bags or storage containers and keep frozen until you are ready to use them. Frozen bananas will keep for up to 3 months.

Green Goodie Smoothie

Spirulina is an antioxidant-rich powder made from blue-green algae. It's highly nutritious and doesn't change the taste of this delicious fruit smoothie. It does, however, make it a beautiful green color.

1 cup unsweetened pineapple juice

1 cup fortified vanilla soymilk or other nondairy milk

1 fresh or frozen banana (see page 100)

10 frozen peach slices

¼ cup fresh or frozen pitted cherries or raspberries

1 tablespoon spirulina powder

2 teaspoons maple syrup (optional)

Ice, as needed (to chill and thicken)

1. Combine all of the ingredients in a blender and process until smooth. Stop the blender occasionally to scrape down the sides of the container and push any unblended fruit into the blades with a rubber spatula.

2. Green Goodie Smoothie is best served immediately. Leftovers may be stored in the refrigerator for up to 1 day or frozen for up to 1 week. Blend the mixture again before serving.

PER SERVING: 122 calories; 1.2 g fat; 0.2 g saturated fat; 9% calories from fat; 0 mg cholesterol; 4.3 g protein; 24.9 g carbohydrate; 16.7 g sugar; 2.3 g fiber; 38 mg sodium; 95 mg calcium; 2.2 mg iron; 46.6 mg vitamin C; 2366 mcg beta-carotene; 1.1 mg vitamin E

Mixed Berry Smoothie

rozen berries in smoothies add fiber, taste, and iciness, not to mention a hefty dose of cancer-fighting compounds.

1 cup frozen mixed berries

1 cup fortified vanilla soymilk or other nondairy milk

1 fresh or frozen banana (see page 100)

2 tablespoons maple syrup (optional)

2 tablespoons calcium-fortified orange juice concentrate

1. Combine all of the ingredients in a blender and process until smooth. Stop the blender occasionally to scrape down the sides of the container and push any unblended fruit into the blades with a rubber spatula.

2. Mixed Berry Smoothie is best served immediately. Leftovers may be stored in the refrigerator for up to 1 day or frozen for up to 1 week. Blend the mixture again before serving.

PER SERVING: 107 calories; 1.4 g fat; 0.2 g saturated fat; 11.5% calories from fat; 0 mg cholesterol; 3.3 g protein; 22.3 g carbohydrate; 12.9 g sugar; 3.7 g fiber; 36 mg sodium; 130 mg calcium; 1 mg iron; 33.1 mg vitamin C; 24 mcg beta-carotene; 1.3 mg vitamin E

Tropical Freeze

uréed frozen fruit makes a wonderful dessert, without the fat or refined sugar in ice cream. Look for frozen mango pieces at your supermarket, or freeze your own using fresh mangoes.

1 orange (preferably navel), peeled

1 cup frozen banana chunks (see page 100)

1 cup frozen mango chunks

½ to 1 cup fortified soymilk or rice milk

1. Cut the orange in half and remove any seeds. Place in a blender along with the banana, mango, and soymilk. Process for 2 to 3 minutes, until thick and completely smooth.

2. Tropical Freeze is best served immediately. Leftovers may be stored in the refrigerator for up to 1 day or frozen for up to 1 week. Blend the mixture again before serving.

PER SERVING: 123 calories; 1 g fat; 0.2 g saturated fat; 7.6% calories from fat; 0 mg cholesterol; 2.7 g protein; 28.7 g carbohydrate; 17.9 g sugar; 3.7 g fiber; 25 mg sodium; 76 mg calcium; 0.7 mg iron; 42.9 mg vitamin C; 289 mcg beta-carotene; 1.3 mg vitamin E

Orange Julius

his beverage is not as sweet as many of the commercially available versions. If you want it sweeter, add a little extra orange juice concentrate.

1 cup fortified soymilk or other nondairy milk

½ cup calcium-fortified orange juice concentrate

½ frozen banana, cut or broken into chunks
(optional; see page 100)

5 ice cubes

1 teaspoon vanilla extract

1. Combine all of the ingredients in a blender and process until smooth and frothy.

2. Orange Julius is best served immediately. Leftovers may be stored in the refrigerator for up to 1 day or frozen for up to 1 week. Blend the mixture again before serving.

PER SERVING: 212 calories; 2.3 g fat; 0.3 g saturated fat; 9.5% calories from fat; 0 mg cholesterol; 6.3 g protein; 42.6 g carbohydrate; 33.7 g sugar; 2.7 g fiber; 73 mg sodium; 502 mg calcium; 1.6 mg iron; 100.9 mg vitamin C; 53 mcg beta-carotene; 2.2 mg vitamin E

Green Tea Smoothie

reen tea contains polyphenolic compounds and catechins, both of which have been found to help fight off cancer.

1½ cups frozen berries
(strawberries, raspberries, or blueberries)

¾ cup fortified soymilk or other nondairy milk

1 frozen banana
(see page 100)

½ cup brewed green tea, cooled or chilled

½ cup cranberry or pomegranate juice

1. Combine all of the ingredients in a blender and process until smooth. Stop the blender occasionally to scrape down the sides of the container and push any unblended fruit into the blades with a rubber spatula.

2. Green Tea Smoothie is best served immediately. Leftovers may be stored in the refrigerator for up to 1 day or frozen for up to 1 week. Blend the mixture again before serving.

PER SERVING: 195 calories; 1.9 g fat; 0.3 g saturated fat; 8.9% calories from fat; 0 mg cholesterol; 4.6 g protein; 43.7 g carbohydrate; 24.8 g sugar; 6 g fiber; 59 mg sodium; 144 mg calcium; 2.4 mg iron; 88.7 mg vitamin C; 64 mcg beta-carotene; 1.9 mg vitamin E

Strawberry Smoothie

Purchase fresh strawberries at the peak of the season, when they're bursting with flavor, to freeze for smoothies. Freezing them is easy: simply remove the stems and place the berries in heavy-duty zipper-lock plastic bags. They'll keep for up to six months. Frozen strawberries are also available at most supermarkets.

1 to 1½ cups fortified soymilk or other nondairy milk

1 cup frozen banana chunks (see page 100)

1 cup frozen strawberries

2 tablespoons apple juice concentrate

½ teaspoon vanilla extract (optional)

1. Combine all of the ingredients in a blender and process until smooth. Stop the blender occasionally to scrape down the sides of the container and push any unblended fruit into the blades with a rubber spatula.

2. Strawberry Smoothie is best served immediately. Leftovers may be stored in the refrigerator for up to 1 day or frozen for up to 1 week. Blend the mixture again before serving.

PER SERVING: 198 calories; 2.6 g fat; 0.4 g saturated fat; 12% calories from fat; 0 mg cholesterol; 5.9 g protein; 41.3 g carbohydrate; 23.7 g sugar; 5.6 g fiber; 76 mg sodium; 175 mg calcium; 2.1 mg iron; 72.3 mg vitamin C; 28 mcg beta-carotene; 2.1 mg vitamin E

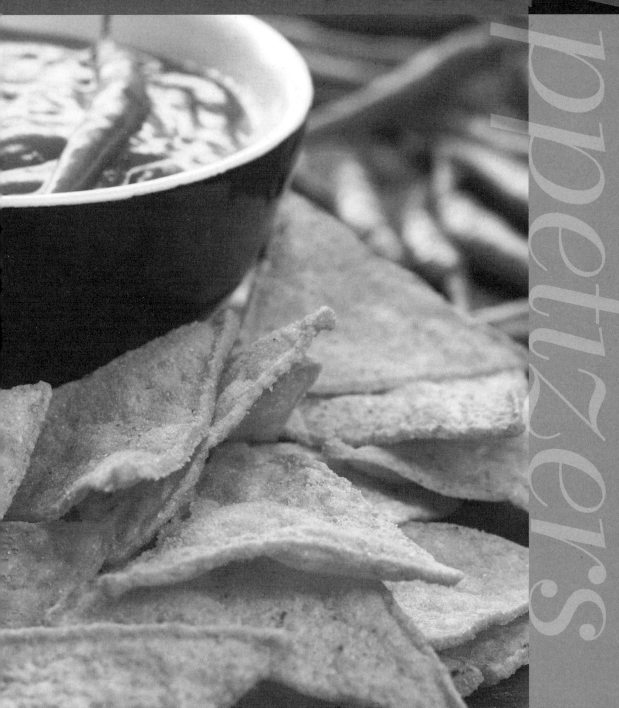

Baked Tortilla Chips

Fat-free baked chips are quick to make using any good-quality corn tortillas. Extra-thin tortillas make especially light and crunchy baked chips.

6 to 8 tablespoons freshly squeezed lime juice

½ teaspoon chili powder

¼ teaspoon ground cumin

12 corn tortillas

¼ teaspoon salt (optional)

1. Preheat the oven to 350 degrees F.

2. Combine the lime juice, chili powder, and cumin in a small pie plate or similar dish. Dip each tortilla into the lime mixture and place them in a stack on a cutting board. Using a chef's knife, cut through the stack, dividing the tortillas into 6 wedges.

3. Arrange the tortillas in a single layer on a wire baking rack or baking sheet and sprinkle with the optional salt. Bake for 10 to 15 minutes, or until the tortillas are crisp and just beginning to brown on the edges. Watch carefully, because they burn quickly. Remove from the oven and let cool.

4. These chips are crispiest when eaten within 1 day. Stored in an air-tight bag or container, leftover Baked Tortilla Chips will keep for up to 1 week.

PER SERVING: 138 calories, 1.6 g fat; 0.2 g saturated fat; 10.6% calories from fat; 0 mg cholesterol; 3.6 g protein; 29.4 g carbohydrate; 1.6 g sugar; 3.5 g fiber; 103 mg sodium; 109 mg calcium; 1 mg iron; 4.9 mg vitamin C; 41 mcg beta-carotene; 0.2 mg vitamin E

Black Bean Dip

This simple bean dip is versatile and virtually fat free. Maintaining a low fat intake is crucial for keeping hormone levels within healthy limits to lower breast and prostate cancer risk. Including the optional cumin will add flavor and antioxidants. Enjoy this dip with raw vegetables, spread it on crackers, or serve it as a sandwich filling.

1½ cups cooked or canned black beans, rinsed and drained

1 cup salsa

½ teaspoon ground cumin
(optional)

1. Combine the beans, salsa, and optional cumin in a food processor or blender and process until smooth. Stop and scrape down the sides of the container with a rubber spatula as needed.

2. Stored in a covered container in the refrigerator, leftover Black Bean Dip will keep for up to 3 days.

PER SERVING: 81 calories; 0.4 g fat; 0.1 g saturated fat; 4.2% calories from fat; 0 mg cholesterol; 4.7 g protein; 15.4 g carbohydrate; 2.7 g sugar; 3.8 g fiber; 280 mg sodium; 47 mg calcium; 1.6 mg iron; 6.4 mg vitamin C; 172 mcg beta-carotene; 0.6 mg vitamin E

Colorful Corn Salsa

orn adds fiber, onions supply allyl sulfides, and tomatoes contribute lycopene to this nutrient-rich salsa—all are cancer-fighting ingredients. Enjoy this dip with baked chips, stuffed in a burrito, or atop a bed of fresh greens.

1 cup fresh or frozen corn kernels

2 medium tomatoes, diced

½ cup diced green bell pepper

½ cup diced orange bell pepper

¼ cup chopped onion

3 to 4 tablespoons freshly squeezed lime juice

3 tablespoons rice vinegar or apple cider vinegar

10 fresh basil leaves, thinly sliced

1. If using fresh corn, blanch it in boiling water for 3 minutes and immediately rinse it under cold water to prevent further cooking. If using frozen corn that isn't thawed completely, either blanch it in boiling water for 2 minutes, drain, and immediately rinse it under cold water, or microwave it until thawed.

2. Combine all of the ingredients in a large bowl and set aside for 15 to 20 minutes to allow the flavors to develop. Serve at room temperature.

3. Stored in a covered container in the refrigerator, leftover Colorful Corn Salsa will keep for up to 3 days.

Note: For the best flavor, remove the desired portion of leftovers and allow it to come to room temperature before serving. If you are preparing this salsa in advance, wait to add the basil until 15 to 20 minutes before serving, as basil quickly oxidizes.

PER SERVING: 13 calories; 0.1 g fat; 0 g saturated fat; 7.5% calories from fat; 0 mg cholesterol; 0.4 g protein; 3 g carbohydrate; 1.1 g sugar; 0.5 g fiber; 1 mg sodium; 4 mg calcium; 0.1 mg iron; 13.6 mg vitamin C; 88 mcg beta-carotene; 0.1 mg vitamin E; 352 mcg lycopene

Creamy Spinach Dip

MAKES 10 TO 12 SERVINGS

 his creamy, high-fiber dip is great for a family gathering or as a dish to pass for a holiday cocktail party. Serve it with raw vegetable pieces or chunks of crusty bread.

1½ cups cooked or canned cannellini beans, rinsed and drained

¼ cup water

2 pounds spinach, chopped and steamed, or 1 package (10 ounces) frozen chopped spinach, thawed and drained

½ cup salsa

1 tablespoon all-purpose seasoning (such as Mrs. Dash, Spike, or Vegit)

1 tablespoon freshly squeezed lemon juice

½ teaspoon salt

1. Mash the beans and water together using a potato masher. Alternatively, process them in a food processor or blender until smooth. Stir in the remaining ingredients and refrigerate for 1 hour before serving.

2. Stored in a covered container in the refrigerator, leftover Creamy Spinach Dip will keep for up to 3 days.

PER SERVING: 61 calories; 0.3 g fat; 0.1 g saturated fat; 3.8% calories from fat; 0 mg cholesterol; 4.2 g protein; 11.3 g carbohydrate; 1 g sugar; 2.9 g fiber; 410 mg sodium; 62 mg calcium; 1.6 mg iron; 3.9 mg vitamin C; 1552 mcg beta-carotene; 1.1 mg vitamin E

Low-Fat Guacamole

T he peas in this guacamole help to lower the fat content, and they are also rich in cancer-fighting fiber. Fiber helps your body get rid of excess cholesterol and cancer-causing compounds that are otherwise reabsorbed into your bloodstream. Despite the addition of peas, this guacamole derives a good portion of its calories from fat. However, the total fat grams and calories are still quite low, and when it is eaten with baked chips as part of a low-fat, plant-based diet, overall fat intake will be within the recommended range.

1 cup canned green peas, rinsed and drained, or 1 cup fresh or frozen green peas

1 ripe avocado

½ cup salsa

3 tablespoons freshly squeezed lemon juice

1 green onion, thinly sliced (optional)

1 tablespoon minced fresh cilantro (optional)

1 garlic clove, minced or pressed

½ teaspoon ground cumin

¼ teaspoon salt

¼ teaspoon ground black pepper

1. If using fresh or frozen peas, blanch them in boiling water for 2 minutes to soften. Drain well and immediately rinse under cold water to prevent further cooking.

2. Cut the avocado in half lengthwise. Twist to separate the halves. Remove the pit and scoop out the flesh with a spoon. For chunky guacamole, mash the avocado and peas together using a potato masher or fork. For a creamier texture, combine the avocado and peas a food processor. Add the salsa, lemon juice, optional green onion, optional cilantro, garlic, and cumin and stir or process until well combined. Season with salt and pepper to taste.

3. Guacamole is best when served the day it is made. To prevent left-over guacamole from turning brown, cover the surface directly with plastic wrap. Stored in a tightly covered container in the refrigerator, Low-Fat Guacamole will keep for up to 1 day.

PER SERVING: 45 calories; 2.7 g fat; 0.4 g saturated fat; 53.5% calories from fat; 0 mg cholesterol; 1.3 g protein; 4.9 g carbohydrate; 1.3 g sugar; 2.1 g fiber; 227 mg sodium; 12 mg calcium; 0.5 mg iron; 6.1 mg vitamin C; 118 mcg beta-carotene; 0.5 mg vitamin E

Mango Salsa

Mango adds a healthful dose of beta-carotene to this refreshing salsa. Beta-carotene is a powerful antioxidant that helps stop free radical damage; it's found in most orange-colored fruits and vegetables. Serve this colorful salsa with Black Bean Chili (page 121) and Baked Tortilla Chips (page 106).

1 large mango, or 5 ounces frozen mango, thawed and diced (about 1 cup)

1 large tomato, seeded (optional) **and diced**

¼ cup minced fresh cilantro

3 tablespoons freshly squeezed lime juice

1 tablespoon minced jalapeño chile, or ½ teaspoon crushed red pepper flakes

¼ teaspoon salt

1. To prepare the fresh mango, peel it and use a sharp paring knife to cut the flesh away from the pit. Cut the flesh into ¼-inch cubes. Alternatively, use the porcupine method (see sidebar). Place the diced mango in a medium mixing bowl.

2. Add all of the remaining ingredients and stir to combine. Let stand 15 minutes to allow the flavors to develop.

3. Stored in a covered container in the refrigerator, leftover Mango Salsa will keep for up to 1 day.

Variation: For Peach Salsa, substitute 1 large peach for the mango.

PER SERVING: 26 calories; 0.2 g fat; 0 g saturated fat; 5.3% calories from fat; 0 mg cholesterol; 0.4 g protein; 6.7 g carbohydrate; 4.8 g sugar; 0.9 g fiber; 77 mg sodium; 6 mg calcium; 0.1 mg iron; 13.5 mg vitamin C; 271 mcg beta-carotene; 0.5 mg vitamin E

How to Dice a Mango Using the Porcupine Method

A mango has two flat sides and two slightly rounded sides. To dice it using the porcupine method, slice the mango once straight down on each of the flat sides with a sharp paring knife, keeping the knife fairly close to the flat seed in the middle (the seed is woody and you will feel when you've hit it with your knife). You should have 2 large, semicircular pieces of mango. For each piece, use the paring knife to gently slice through the mango flesh in a crisscross fashion without cutting through the peel. Then press the piece inside out so it looks like a porcupine. Carefully cut the cubes off of the peel using the paring knife. Repeat this process with the remaining portions. Then carefully slice and dice any ripe chunks from the middle section of the fruit that are still clinging to the seed.

Potato Boats with Spinach Stuffing

This is a delicious way to dress up leftover baked or steamed potatoes. These go particularly well with Black Bean Chili (page 121). This recipe contains millet, a grain that is rich in B vitamins and iron.

1½ cups water

¼ cup millet, rinsed and drained

4 medium russet potatoes

2 pounds fresh spinach, chopped, or 1 package (10 ounces) **frozen chopped spinach, thawed and drained**

2 tablespoons raw cashews

1 teaspoon salt

¼ teaspoon ground black pepper

¼ teaspoon ground nutmeg

1 tablespoon toasted sesame seeds (optional)

1. Place 1 cup of the water and all of the millet in a small saucepan and bring to a boil. Lower the heat, cover, and cook for 30 to 45 minutes (the longer cooking time will make the millet creamier), or until all of the water is absorbed. Set aside.

2. Bake, microwave, or steam the potatoes until they are tender when pierced with a knife. When cool enough to handle, carefully cut the potatoes in half lengthwise. Scoop out the flesh into a bowl, leaving a ¼-inch-thick shell. Set the flesh and shells aside.

3. Steam the spinach until tender. Drain well.

4. Combine the millet, cashews, salt, pepper, and nutmeg in a blender with the remaining ½ cup of water. Process on high speed until completely smooth, about 2 minutes, stopping the blender occasionally to scrape down the sides of the container with a rubber spatula.

5. Transfer the potato flesh to a skillet and use a spoon to break it into bite-size chunks. Add the spinach and warm over medium heat, stirring often. When hot, stir in the millet mixture. Cook over medium-high heat for 2 to 3 minutes to heat through and thicken slightly. Scoop into the reserved potato shells and sprinkle with the optional sesame seeds before serving.

6. Stored in a covered container in the refrigerator, leftover Potato Boats with Spinach Stuffing will keep for up to 2 days. Reheat them in the oven or microwave before serving.

PER SERVING: 124 calories; 1.5 g fat; 0.3 g saturated fat; 10.8% calories from fat; 0 mg cholesterol; 4.1 g protein; 24.8 g carbohydrate; 1.3 g sugar; 3.4 g fiber; 327 mg sodium; 51 mg calcium; 1.7 mg iron; 8.8 mg vitamin C; 1700 mcg beta-carotene; 0.9 mg vitamin E

Roasted Red Pepper Hummus

S pread hummus on whole wheat pita bread or serve it as a dip for vegetables. This version is lower in fat than most commercial brands, which is important when it comes to reducing hormone-dependent cancer risk and keeping your immune system operating smoothly. Keep whole wheat pita and cut veggies on hand for a quick meal or snack.

1½ cups cooked or canned chickpeas, rinsed and drained

½ cup roasted red bell peppers packed in water, drained

3 green onions, sliced

¼ cup freshly squeezed lemon juice

1 tablespoon tahini

3 garlic cloves, minced or pressed

1 teaspoon ground cumin

½ teaspoon ground black pepper

¼ cup bean cooking liquid or vegetable broth (optional)

1. Place the chickpeas, red peppers, green onions, lemon juice, tahini, garlic, cumin, and pepper in a food processor or blender and process until smooth. Add the bean cooking liquid as needed to facilitate processing and achieve a smoother consistency.

2. Stored in a covered container in the refrigerator, leftover Roasted Red Pepper Hummus will keep for up to 3 days.

PER SERVING: 80 calories; 2.1 g fat; 0.3 g saturated fat; 23.3% calories from fat; 0 mg cholesterol; 3.9 g protein; 12.5 g carbohydrate; 1.4 g sugar; 2.8 g fiber; 32 mg sodium; 36 mg calcium; 1.6 mg iron; 23.5 mg vitamin C; 299 mcg beta-carotene; 0.4 mg vitamin E

Roasted Sweet Potato Wedges

Once you try this version of "fries," you'll be hooked! They're loaded with cancer-fighting beta-carotene, and baking them eliminates any added fat.

2 medium sweet potatoes (unpeeled), **washed and cut into wedges**

¼ teaspoon salt

¼ teaspoon ground cumin

¼ teaspoon garlic powder

⅛ teaspoon ground cinnamon

⅛ teaspoon ground black pepper

1. Preheat the oven to 450 degrees F. Lightly mist a baking sheet with vegetable oil spray.
2. Combine the sweet potatoes, salt, cumin, garlic powder, cinnamon, and black pepper in a zipper-lock plastic bag. Seal the bag and shake it until the sweet potatoes are evenly coated.
3. Arrange the sweet potatoes in a single layer on the prepared baking sheet. Bake for 10 minutes, turn the wedges over, and bake for 10 minutes longer, or until very tender.
4. Roasted Sweet Potato Wedges will be the crispiest when served soon after roasting. Stored in a covered container in the refrigerator, leftover Roasted Sweet Potato Wedges will keep for up to 3 days.

PER SERVING: 53 calories; 0.1 g fat; 0 g saturated fat; 2.1% calories from fat; 0 mg cholesterol; 1.2 g protein; 12.1 g total carbohydrate; 4.8 g sugar; 2 g fiber; 106 mg sodium; 24 mg calcium; 0.5 mg iron; 11.3 mg vitamin C; 6561 mcg beta-carotene; 0.4 mg vitamin E

Soybean Snacks (Edamame)

Edamame is the Japanese term for young green soybeans. If you've never tasted this delicious and highly nutritious snack, you're in for a real treat. Edamame is sold fresh in Asian markets and some specialty stores. It is available either shelled or unshelled in the frozen food section of most supermarkets and natural food stores. Soybeans are higher in fat than any other bean, so enjoy this snack along with a low-fat meal to minimize your overall fat intake.

6 cups water

1 pound unshelled edamame

½ teaspoon salt (optional)

1. Bring the water to a boil in a large pot. Add the edamame and return to a boil. Lower the heat slightly, cover, and cook for about 8 minutes, until the beans are just tender. Drain and toss with the optional salt.

2. Transfer to a serving bowl and provide a plate for the discarded pods.

3. Stored in a covered container in the refrigerator, leftover Soybean Snacks will keep for up to 3 days.

PER SERVING: 100 calories; 4.5 g fat; 0.5 g saturated fat; 40.9% calories from fat; 0 mg cholesterol; 8.8 g protein; 7.8 g carbohydrate; 1 g sugar; 3 g fiber; 10 mg sodium; 103 mg calcium; 1.8 mg iron; 12.1 mg vitamin C; 67 mcg beta-carotene; 0 mg vitamin E

Stuffed Mushrooms

S tuffed Mushrooms are a great party food, because they can be made in advance and served at room temperature or heated just before serving. Mushrooms are rich in fiber, which helps boost immune strength.

¾ cup water

¼ cup millet, rinsed

5 ounces chopped fresh spinach, steamed, or 1 package (10 ounces) frozen chopped spinach, thawed and drained

2 tablespoons raw cashews, or 2 teaspoons cashew butter

2 teaspoons onion powder

¾ teaspoon salt

½ teaspoon garlic powder

1 tablespoon soy sauce

1 tablespoon balsamic vinegar

2 garlic cloves, minced or pressed

20 large button or cremini mushrooms, cleaned and stems removed

2 green onions, thinly sliced

1 teaspoon dried basil

1 tablespoon toasted or raw sesame seeds

1. Combine the water and millet in a small saucepan and bring to a boil. Lower the heat, cover, and simmer for about 30 minutes, or until all of the water is absorbed.

2. Place the spinach in a colander and press out as much liquid as possible.

3. Combine the millet, cashews, onion powder, salt, and garlic powder in a blender and process on high for about 2 minutes, or until the mixture is very smooth. Stop the blender occasionally to scrape down sides of the container with a rubber spatula. Set aside.

4. Warm the soy sauce and vinegar in a nonstick skillet. When the mixture begins to bubble, add the garlic and cook and stir over medium heat for 1 minute, or until slightly softened. Add the mushrooms, top sides down. Cover and cook over medium-high heat for 3 minutes, or until the tops are browned. Turn the mushrooms over and cook for 3 minutes longer. Remove from the pan and set aside.

5. Without washing the pan, add the spinach, green onions, and basil. Cook and stir over medium heat for about 2 minutes, or until the spinach is very dry. Add the millet mixture and sesame seeds and continue to cook, stirring constantly, until the mixture is thick and heated through. Spoon into the mushroom caps and serve warm or at room temperature.

6. Stored in a covered container in the refrigerator, leftover Stuffed Mushrooms will keep for up to 2 days. To reheat the mushrooms, place them in a baking dish and warm them in a preheated 350 degree F oven for about 12 minutes.

PER SERVING: 127 calories; 3.6 g fat; 0.6 g saturated fat; 25.4% calories from fat; 0 mg cholesterol; 5.9 g protein; 20.1 g carbohydrate; 1.6 g sugar; 4.8 g fiber; 577 mg sodium; 95 mg calcium; 3 mg iron; 5.9 mg vitamin C; 2750 mcg beta-carotene; 1.4 mg vitamin E

Texas Caviar

This colorful and crunchy "caviar" is full of fiber, very low in fat, and cholesterol free, making it a wonderful dip for reducing cancer risk. Scoop it up with Baked Tortilla Chips (page 106) or wedges of whole-grain pita bread.

½ cup bulgur

¼ teaspoon salt

1 cup boiling water

1½ cups cooked or canned black-eyed peas, rinsed and drained

2 tomatoes, finely chopped

1 green bell pepper, finely chopped

3 green onions, finely chopped

¼ cup minced fresh cilantro

3 tablespoons freshly squeezed lime juice

1 to 2 chipotle chiles in adobo sauce, minced, or ¼ teaspoon crushed red pepper flakes

1 to 2 teaspoons adobo sauce (from the chiles; optional)

½ teaspoon ground cumin

¼ teaspoon ground coriander

1. Combine the bulgur and salt in a large bowl. Stir in the boiling water, cover, and let stand for about 25 minutes, or until the bulgur is tender. Drain off any excess water.

2. Transfer the bulgur to a large mixing bowl. Add all of the remaining ingredients and stir until well combined. Taste and adjust the salt, lime juice, and adobo sauce if needed. Chill for at least 1 hour before serving.

3. Stored in a covered container in the refrigerator, leftover Texas Caviar will keep for up to 3 days.

PER SERVING: 43 calories; 0.2 g fat; 0.1 g saturated fat; 5% calories from fat; 0 mg cholesterol; 2.2 g protein; 8.6 g carbohydrate; 1 g sugar; 2.1 g fiber; 134 mg sodium; 13 mg calcium; 0.8 mg iron; 10.1 mg vitamin C; 117 mcg beta-carotene; 0.2 mg vitamin E

Veggies in a Blanket

This party food is simple to prepare. It can be made with your favorite bean spread and fresh vegetables, and kids just love them. Take a whole wrap as a to-go lunch—it's filling and loaded with cancer-fighting fiber and many health-promoting nutrients.

1 cup low-fat hummus or bean spread

8 whole wheat tortillas

4 carrots, grated

8 lettuce leaves, 1 cup baby spinach, or 5 ounces alfalfa or bean sprouts

1. Spread the hummus thinly on the tortillas. Add the carrots and lettuce. Roll up each tortilla and secure with 5 evenly placed toothpicks. Slice into 5 individual rolls per tortilla (one toothpick per roll).

2. Serve Veggies in a Blanket immediately or cover tightly and store in the refrigerator for several hours. Prior to serving, bring the rolls to room temperature for the best flavor. Do not store the rolls longer than 1 day, as the tortillas and lettuce will become soggy.

Variation: Add thin sticks of cucumber or red bell pepper before rolling.

PER SERVING: 122 calories; 2.8 g fat; 0.3 g saturated fat; 18% calories from fat; 0 mg cholesterol; 5 g protein; 20.6 g carbohydrate; 1.5 g sugar; 4.9 g fiber; 251 mg sodium; 27 mg calcium; 2 mg iron; 2.1 mg vitamin C; 1424 mcg beta-carotene; 0.4 mg vitamin E

White Bean Spread with Sun-Dried Tomatoes

This luscious spread uses no added fat. The sun-dried tomatoes give it a wonderful smoky flavor and add the cancer-fighting antioxidant lycopene. Spread it on low-fat crusty bread or use it as a dip for baked pita chips.

6 sun-dried tomatoes (not packed in oil)

1 cup boiling water

1½ cups cooked or canned great northern beans, rinsed and drained

1 teaspoon finely chopped fresh rosemary, or 1 teaspoon dried rosemary, crumbled

1 teaspoon freshly squeezed lemon juice

2 garlic cloves, minced or pressed, or ½ teaspoon garlic powder

½ teaspoon salt

½ teaspoon dried sage

½ cup bean cooking liquid or vegetable broth (optional)

1. Place the sun-dried tomatoes in a heatproof bowl and pour the boiling water over them. Let soak until softened, about 10 minutes. Drain, thinly slice, and set aside.

2. Combine the beans, rosemary, lemon juice, garlic, salt, and sage in a food processor and process until smooth. If desired, add some or all of the bean cooking liquid for a creamier texture. Stir in the sun-dried tomatoes. Taste and add more salt or lemon juice if needed.

3. Stored in a covered container in the refrigerator, leftover White Bean Spread with Sun-Dried Tomatoes will keep for up to 3 days.

PER SERVING: 74 calories; 0.2 g fat; 0.1 g saturated fat; 2.9% calories from fat; 0 mg cholesterol; 5 g protein; 13.6 g carbohydrate; 0.9 g sugar; 3.3 g fiber; 381 mg sodium; 49 mg calcium; 2 mg iron; 1.4 mg vitamin C; 11 mcg beta-carotene; 0.5 mg vitamin E; 688 mcg lycopene

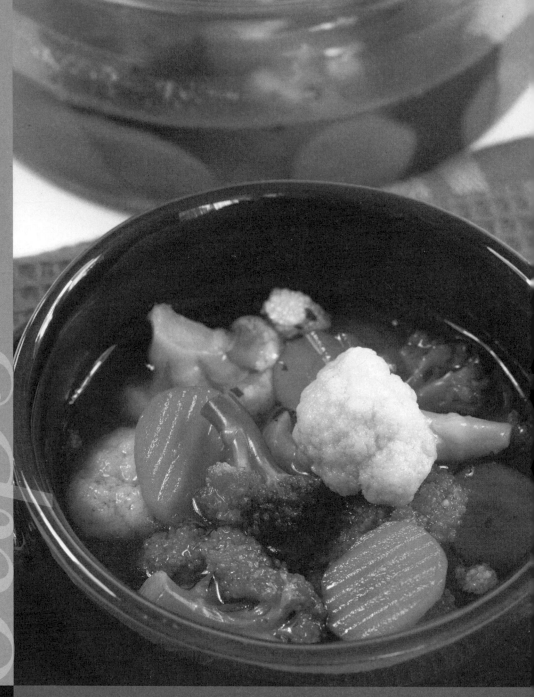

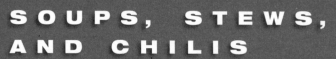

SOUPS, STEWS, AND CHILIS

Soups

Black Bean Chili

apsaicin, the active compound in hot chiles, can help destroy cancer cells. Capsaicin is most concentrated in chile seeds. This recipe is quick to prepare and delicious served with brown rice and a green salad. It can also be used as a burrito filling. If you enjoy a lot of heat, add more chiles.

½ cup water

½ onion, diced

½ green bell pepper, diced

4 garlic cloves, minced or pressed

1 teaspoon dried oregano

1 teaspoon ground cumin

3 cups cooked or canned black beans, rinsed and drained

1 can (15 ounces) diced tomatoes, undrained, or 1½ cups chopped fresh tomatoes

½ cup bean cooking liquid or vegetable broth

½ cup frozen corn, thawed, or canned corn, drained

1 to 2 canned chipotle chiles in adobo sauce, or ¼ teaspoon crushed red pepper flakes

1 teaspoon adobo sauce (from the chipotle chiles; optional)

Salt

1. Heat the water in a large soup pot. Add the onion, bell pepper, garlic, oregano, and cumin. Cook and stir over medium heat for about 5 minutes, or until the onion is soft.

2. Add the beans, tomatoes, bean cooking liquid, corn, chiles, and optional adobo sauce, cover, and simmer, stirring occasionally, for about 20 minutes, or until the mixture has thickened and the flavors have blended. Season with salt to taste.

3. Stored in a covered container in the refrigerator, leftover Black Bean Chili will keep for up to 3 days.

PER SERVING: 259 calories; 1.3 g fat; 0.3 g saturated fat; 4.6% calories from fat; 0 mg cholesterol; 14.6 g protein; 50.3 g carbohydrate; 9.2 g sugar; 11.4 g fiber; 752 mg sodium; 157 mg calcium; 5.5 mg iron; 27.7 mg vitamin C; 138 mcg beta-carotene; 1.2 mg vitamin E

Cream of Broccoli Soup

B roccoli contains sulforaphane, a powerful antioxidant that has been shown to be particularly beneficial against breast and prostate cancer. New research suggests that the cancer-protective effects of sulforaphane may last for days. This creamy soup is a delicious way to serve broccoli, a nutritional powerhouse, to children, and the addition of chickpeas makes it a one-dish meal.

4 cups water or vegetable broth

1 large potato (preferably russet), **unpeeled, scrubbed, and cut into chunks**

1 onion, diced

3 whole garlic cloves, peeled

1 teaspoon whole celery seeds

1 teaspoon dried thyme

½ teaspoon dried marjoram

¼ teaspoon ground turmeric

¼ teaspoon ground black pepper

1½ cups cooked or canned chickpeas, rinsed and drained

¼ cup bean cooking liquid, vegetable broth, or water

4 cups broccoli florets

1½ teaspoons salt, as needed

1. Combine the water, potato, onion, garlic, celery seeds, thyme, marjoram, turmeric, and pepper in a large soup pot. Place over medium heat, cover, and simmer for about 20 minutes, or until the vegetables are tender.

2. Stir in the chickpeas and the bean cooking liquid. Remove from the heat and let cool slightly. Transfer to a blender and process in several batches, filling the blender container no more than half full for each batch. Hold the lid on tightly and start the blender on the lowest speed. Process for 1 to 2 minutes, or until the mixture is completely smooth.

3. Return the blended soup to the pot and stir in the broccoli and 1 teaspoon of the salt. Cover and simmer for 5 to 10 minutes, or until the broccoli is fork-tender. Taste and add the remaining ½ teaspoon of salt if desired.

4. Stored in a covered container in the refrigerator, leftover Cream of Broccoli Soup will keep for up to 3 days.

PER SERVING: 151 calories; 1.5 g fat; 0.2 g saturated fat; 9.1% calories from fat; 0 mg cholesterol; 7.4 g protein; 29.1 g carbohydrate; 2.4 g sugar; 6.5 g fiber; 475 mg sodium; 75 mg calcium; 3.2 mg iron; 32 mg vitamin C; 396 mcg beta-carotene; 1 mg vitamin E

Creamy Root Soup

This soup is made with a variety of root vegetables and supplies an assortment of cancer-fighting antioxidants to help prevent free radical damage. Rutabaga is a type of cruciferous vegetable; it contains the antioxidants beta-carotene and sulforaphane, which are particularly important for protecting against breast cancer. This recipe also includes a variety of healthful spices, such as turmeric and curry powder, which contain the cancer-fighting compound curcumin.

3½ to 4 cups water or vegetable broth

1 large onion, diced

½ teaspoon ground ginger

½ teaspoon ground cumin

½ teaspoon ground turmeric

⅛ teaspoon crushed red pepper flakes or cayenne

1 medium rutabaga, peeled and diced

1 large russet potato, unpeeled, scrubbed, and diced

1 large sweet potato, unpeeled, scrubbed, and diced

2 large carrots, diced or cut into half-moons

1½ teaspoons salt

4 cups spinach, chopped

1. Heat ½ cup of the water in a large soup pot. Add the onion and cook and stir over high heat for about 5 minutes, or until soft and translucent. Add the ginger, cumin, turmeric, and red pepper flakes and cook and stir for 2 minutes.

2. Stir in 3 cups of the remaining water and the rutabaga, russet potato, sweet potato, carrots, and salt. Cover and simmer, stirring occasionally, for about 30 minutes, or until the vegetables are tender and the soup has thickened.

3. Stir in the spinach and simmer until it is just tender, about 5 minutes. If desired, add the remaining ½ cup of water for a thinner soup.

4. Stored in a covered container in the refrigerator, leftover Creamy Root Soup will keep for up to 3 days.

PER SERVING: 70 calories; 0.3 g fat; 0.1 g saturated fat; 3.3% calories from fat; 0 mg cholesterol; 2 g protein; 16 g carbohydrate; 3.8 g sugar; 2.9 g fiber; 386 mg sodium; 55 mg calcium; 1.5 mg iron; 16.6 mg vitamin C; 3767 mcg beta-carotene; 0.6 mg vitamin E

Curried Sweet Potato Soup

Eating blended soup is a great way to get in loads of nutritious vegetables. One serving of this soup provides more than your daily recommended intake of beta-carotene, which has been deemed one of the most significant nutrients for improving breast cancer survival.

4¼ cups vegetable broth

1 cup diced onion

2 teaspoons curry powder

5 cups peeled and chopped sweet potatoes

1 cup water

1 cup plus 6 tablespoons plain nondairy yogurt

½ cup minced fresh cilantro (optional)

1. Heat ¼ cup of the broth in a large soup pot over medium-high heat. Add the onion and curry powder and cook and stir for 2 minutes. Add the remaining 4 cups of broth, the sweet potatoes, and the water. Cook for 30 minutes, or until the sweet potatoes are tender. Remove from the heat and let cool slightly.

2. Transfer one-third of the sweet potato mixture to a blender and process until smooth. Repeat the procedure with the remaining sweet potato mixture, processing it in batches. Return the blended mixture to the pot and bring to a boil. Remove from the heat, add 1 cup of the yogurt, and stir until blended.

3. Top each serving with 1 tablespoon of the remaining yogurt and garnish with the optional cilantro.

4. Stored in a covered container in the refrigerator, leftover Curried Sweet Potato Soup will keep for up to 3 days.

PER SERVING: 177 calories; 1.4 g fat; 0.2 g saturated fat; 7.1% calories from fat; 0 mg cholesterol; 4.9 g protein; 37.5 g total carbohydrate; 12.9 g sugar; 4.5 g fiber; 770 mg sodium; 128 mg calcium; 1.8 mg iron; 25.4 mg vitamin C; 13266 mcg beta-carotene; 1.3 mg vitamin E

Latin Seitan Stew

The bell peppers in this dish add vitamin C, an antioxidant that plays an important role in boosting the immune system. This dish also contains seitan, a fat-free, high-protein food made from wheat gluten, which is often used as a meat alternative. Seitan can be found in natural food stores and well-stocked supermarkets.

2 cups vegetable broth

1 red bell pepper, diced

1 green bell pepper, diced

1 onion, diced

5 garlic cloves, minced or pressed

3 celery stalks, diced

½ cup mashed or blended tomatoes

2 cups cut green beans, in 1-inch pieces

4 carrots, diced

2 bay leaves

2 teaspoons dried thyme

2 teaspoons dried rosemary

8 cups water

10 small red or white potatoes, cut into 2-inch cubes

¾ cup millet or quinoa, rinsed and drained

3 cups diced tomatoes

2 tablespoons tamari

2 teaspoons ground cumin

1 teaspoon salt

1 package (8 ounces) seitan, cut into 1-inch pieces

½ cup red wine or nonalcoholic alternative

1½ cups green peas

1 to 3 tablespoons cornstarch or kuzu dissolved in 2 to 6 tablespoons red wine or water (optional)

1. Place ¼ cup of the vegetable broth in a large soup pot. Add the red and green bell peppers, onion, and garlic. Cook and stir over medium-high heat for 2 minutes.

2. Add the celery and mashed tomatoes and cook for 2 to 3 minutes. Add the green beans, carrots, bay leaves, thyme, and rosemary. Cook and stir for 3 minutes.

3. Add the remaining 1¾ cups of vegetable broth and all of the water, potatoes, and millet and bring to a boil. Stir in the diced tomatoes, tamari, cumin, and salt. Cook over medium heat for 15 minutes.

4. Stir in the seitan and wine. Cook for 10 to 15 minutes, or until the millet is tender. Add the peas and cook for 5 minutes longer.

5. If the broth is not thick enough, dissolve the cornstarch, 1 tablespoon at a time, in 2 tablespoons of red wine. Stir this mixture into the simmering soup. Add additional tablespoons of cornstarch dissolved in 2 tablespoons of red wine until the desired thickness is reached.

6. Stored in a covered container in the refrigerator, Latin Seitan Stew will keep for up to 3 days.

Note: If you are unable to find seitan, use 1 cup of cooked lentils instead.

PER SERVING: 335 calories; 1.8 g fat; 0.3 g saturated fat; 4.8% calories from fat; 0 mg cholesterol; 15 g protein; 67.7 g carbohydrate; 10.2 g sugar; 11 g fiber; 925 mg sodium; 120 mg calcium; 6.2 mg iron; 77.5 mg vitamin C; 3661 mcg beta-carotene; 1.4 mg vitamin E

Lentil Artichoke Stew

The artichokes in this stew add fiber, vitamin C, and folate. This aromatic and tasty Middle Eastern dish is great served alone or over brown rice or pasta. Using fire-roasted tomatoes is not essential, but they will give the stew a delicious smoky flavor.

¼ cup vegetable broth

1 onion, diced

2 large garlic cloves, minced or pressed

2 teaspoons ground cumin

1 teaspoon ground coriander

2 cups water

1 cup dried red lentils

1 bay leaf

2 cans (24 ounces each) chopped fire-roasted tomatoes, undrained, or 6 cups chopped fresh tomatoes plus 1 cup tomato juice

1 can (15 ounces) water-packed artichoke hearts, drained and quartered, or 1 package (9 ounces) frozen artichoke hearts, thawed and quartered

3 to 4 tablespoons freshly squeezed lemon juice

¼ teaspoon crushed red pepper flakes (optional)

¼ teaspoon salt

¼ teaspoon ground black pepper

1. Heat the broth in a large soup pot. Add the onion and cook and stir over medium heat for about 5 minutes, until translucent.

2. Add the garlic, cumin, and coriander and cook for 2 minutes, stirring frequently.

3. Add the water, lentils, and bay leaf and bring to a boil.

4. Lower the heat and add the tomatoes and their liquid, the artichoke hearts, lemon juice, and optional red pepper flakes. Simmer for about 20 minutes, or until the lentils are tender. Remove and discard the bay leaf. Season with salt and pepper to taste.

5. Stored in a covered container in the refrigerator, leftover Lentil Artichoke Stew will keep for up to 3 days.

Note: If red lentils are unavailable, green lentils can be substituted. However, because green lentils will not cook properly in acidic foods, such as tomatoes and lemon juice, you will need to cook them in water or vegetable broth until tender prior to adding them to the stew.

PER SERVING: 176 calories; 1 g fat; 0.1 g saturated fat; 4.9% calories from fat; 0 mg cholesterol; 11.7 g protein; 34.3 g carbohydrate; 7.5 g sugar; 10 g fiber; 560 mg sodium; 123 mg calcium; 6.3 mg iron; 28.6 mg vitamin C; 238 mcg beta-carotene; 1.8 mg vitamin E

Lentil and Brown Rice Soup

This hearty soup is high in plant protein and beneficial fiber, which will help you to feel full longer and make it easier for you to maintain a healthy weight. For a satisfying meal, serve this soup with whole-grain bread and a cucumber salad.

12 cups water or vegetable broth

1 cup dried brown or green lentils

1 cup short-grain brown rice

1 cup diced onion

1 cup minced fresh parsley

6 garlic cloves, minced

1 teaspoon dried oregano

1 teaspoon dried thyme

½ teaspoon ground black pepper

¼ teaspoon whole celery seeds

¼ teaspoon ground cinnamon

¼ teaspoon salt

1. Bring the water to a boil in a large soup pot. Add the lentils, rice, onion, parsley, garlic, oregano, thyme, pepper, celery seeds, and cinnamon. Lower the heat, cover loosely, and simmer, stirring occasionally, for about 45 minutes, or until the lentils and rice are tender.

2. Season with the salt to taste.

3. Stored in a covered container in the refrigerator, leftover Lentil and Brown Rice Soup will keep for up to 3 days.

PER SERVING: 173 calories; 1.1 g fat; 0.2 g saturated fat; 5.6% calories from fat; 0 mg cholesterol; 8.5 g protein; 33.4 g carbohydrate; 1 g sugar; 7 g fiber; 158 mg sodium; 43 mg calcium; 3.3 mg iron; 12.2 mg vitamin C; 390 mcg beta-carotene; 0.2 mg vitamin E

Miso Soup with Shiitake Mushrooms

Miso, also known as soybean paste, is a traditional Japanese food. It is most commonly used for making miso soup, which is served with every meal in Japan. There are different types of miso, each with a distinctive, characteristic flavor. This recipe uses white miso, which has a mellow, slightly sweet flavor. Miso is available at natural food stores and Asian markets; it can also be purchased online. The shiitake mushrooms in this soup add vitamin D, an important nutrient for cancer prevention.

5 cups vegetable broth

1 ounce dried shiitake mushrooms

½ pound firm tofu, cut into ¼-inch cubes

1 sheet nori, cut into 1-inch squares

2 to 3 teaspoons peeled and grated fresh ginger

2 cups small broccoli florets

1 cup julienned or grated carrots

3 to 4 tablespoons white miso

1. Pour the broth into a large soup pot and bring to a boil. Remove from the heat, add the mushrooms, cover, and let stand for 20 minutes, or until the mushrooms have softened. Remove the mushrooms from the broth with a slotted spoon. Cut off and discard the mushroom stems. Thinly slice the caps and set aside.

2. Add the tofu, nori, and ginger to the broth. Bring to a simmer and cook for 3 minutes. Add the mushrooms, broccoli, and carrots. Cover and simmer for 1 minute, just until the broccoli turns bright green.

3. Transfer 1 cup of the broth to a measuring cup and stir in the miso with a fork until it is completely dissolved. Pour the dissolved miso into the soup and stir until it is well incorporated. Serve immediately.

4. Stored in a covered container in the refrigerator, leftover Miso Soup with Shiitake Mushrooms will keep for up to 3 days.

Note: Do not boil the soup after the miso has been added, as high heat will destroy the beneficial enzymes in the miso.

PER SERVING: 92 calories; 2.8 g fat; 0.4 g saturated fat; 27.2% calories from fat; 0 mg cholesterol; 6.5 g protein; 12.8 g carbohydrate; 5.9 g sugar; 2.8 g fiber; 1167 mg sodium; 92 mg calcium; 1.4 mg iron; 13.4 mg vitamin C; 2314 mcg beta-carotene; 0.8 mg vitamin E

Mushroom Barley Soup

This soup takes just minutes to make if you have cooked barley on hand. Because it is very low in fat, it helps the immune system recognize and destroy cancer cells. All fats, including healthful vegetable fats, should be kept to a minimum when it comes to cancer prevention and survival.

⅔ cup water

⅓ cup pearl barley, regular or quick-cooking

2 cups fortified plain rice milk

2 tablespoons barley flour

1 can (4 ounces) mushrooms, undrained, or 6 fresh mushrooms, quartered

¼ teaspoon garlic powder

¼ teaspoon salt

Pinch of dried marjoram

Pinch of dried sage

Pinch of dried thyme

Pinch of dried dill weed

1. To cook the barley, bring the water and barley to a boil in a medium saucepan. Lower the heat, cover, and cook until all of the water has been absorbed, about 30 minutes for regular barley or 10 minutes for quick-cooking barley.

2. Place the rice milk and flour in a blender and process on high speed for a few seconds. Add the cooked barley and process on high speed for about 10 seconds, just until the barley is coarsely chopped. Add the mushrooms and their liquid and process very briefly, just until they are coarsely chopped.

3. Transfer the blended mixture to a medium saucepan and stir in the garlic powder, salt, marjoram, sage, thyme, and dill weed. Cook over medium heat, stirring often, for about 5 minutes, or until the soup is hot and slightly thickened.

4. Stored in a covered container in the refrigerator, leftover Mushroom Barley Soup will keep for up to 3 days.

Note: If you prefer, omit the water and barley and substitute 1 cup cooked barley.

PER SERVING: 172 calories; 1.7 g fat; 0.2 g saturated fat; 8.9% calories from fat; 0 mg cholesterol; 3.2 g protein; 36.7 g carbohydrate; 9 g sugar; 4.1 g fiber; 350 mg sodium; 213 mg calcium; 1 mg iron; 0.9 mg vitamin C; 9 mcg beta-carotene; 1.2 mg vitamin E

Portuguese Kale and Potato Soup

This recipe calls for substantially fewer hot chiles than would be used by a traditional Portuguese cook. If you want to make a spicier version, double the chipotle chiles and throw in some jalapeños for good measure. Chipotle chiles in adobo sauce can be found in the Mexican food section of well-stocked supermarkets. They are also available at Mexican grocery stores and from online retailers. This recipe is abundant in garlic. When crushed, garlic can provide powerful cancer-protective effects.

4 cups water or vegetable broth

1 onion, diced

10 garlic cloves, minced or pressed

1 chipotle chile in adobo sauce, seeded and finely chopped, or ⅛ teaspoon crushed red pepper flakes

2 potatoes (preferably russet), peeled and diced

½ teaspoon salt (optional)

4 cups stemmed and finely chopped kale

1 cup crushed tomatoes or tomato sauce

6 ounces vegetarian sausage

1. Heat ½ cup of the water in a large pot. Add the onion, garlic, and chile and cook over high heat, stirring often, for 3 to 5 minutes, or until the onion is soft.

2. Add the remaining 3½ cups of water, the potatoes, and optional salt. Bring to a simmer, cover, and cook, stirring occasionally, for about 20 minutes, or until the potatoes are tender when pierced with a knife.

3. Stir in the kale and crushed tomatoes. Cover and cook for about 5 minutes, or until the kale is tender.

4. Crumble the vegetarian sausage into the soup, stir to mix, and heat until the soup is steaming and the sausage is heated through.

5. Stored in a covered container in the refrigerator, leftover Portuguese Kale and Potato soup will keep for up to 3 days.

Note: This recipe is delicious served over Garlic Mashed Potatoes (page 177).

PER SERVING: 91 calories; 1.5 g fat; 0.2 g saturated fat; 14.7% calories from fat; 0 mg cholesterol; 5.8 g protein; 15.1 g carbohydrate; 2.1 g sugar; 2.3 g fiber; 260 mg sodium; 62 mg calcium; 1.3 mg iron; 23 mg vitamin C; 3077 mcg beta-carotene; 0.7 mg vitamin E

Sweet-and-Sour Vegetable Stew

This colorful stew is full of a variety of cancer-fighting phytochemicals (plant compounds). For example, the tomatoes contain lycopene, which has proven to be effective in prostate cancer prevention and survival. Serve it with Braised Kale (page 173) and aromatic rice (such as basmati or jasmine) or couscous.

½ cup water or vegetable broth

1 onion, diced

1 jewel or garnet yam, peeled (if desired) and cut into ½-inch cubes

1 large carrot, diced or cut into rounds or half-moons

1 cup sliced celery

1 can (15 ounces) diced tomatoes, undrained, or 1½ cups chopped fresh tomatoes

1½ cups cooked or canned chickpeas, rinsed and drained

1 can (8 ounces) crushed pineapple packed in juice, or 1 cup crushed fresh pineapple with juice

1 cup chopped roasted red bell peppers

½ cup bean cooking liquid, vegetable broth, or water

½ cup minced fresh cilantro

1 tablespoon minced jalapeño chile, or ½ teaspoon crushed red pepper flakes

1 teaspoon peeled and minced fresh ginger, or ¼ teaspoon ground ginger

1 teaspoon curry powder

¼ teaspoon ground cinnamon

¼ teaspoon ground coriander

1. Heat the water in a large soup pot. Add the onion, yam, carrot, and celery. Cook over medium heat, stirring often, for about 7 minutes, or until the vegetables begin to soften.

2. Add all of the remaining ingredients, cover, and cook, stirring occasionally, for 15 to 20 minutes, or until the vegetables are tender.

3. Stored in a covered container in the refrigerator, leftover Sweet-and-Sour Vegetable Stew will keep for up to 3 days.

PER SERVING: 121 calories; 1.2 g fat; 0.1 g saturated fat; 9.1% calories from fat; 0 mg cholesterol; 4.8 g protein; 24.7 g carbohydrate; 9.9 g sugar; 4.7 g fiber; 145 mg sodium; 62 mg calcium; 2.1 mg iron; 53.6 mg vitamin C; 3517 mcg beta-carotene; 1.3 mg vitamin E; 1435 mcg lycopene

Three Bean Chili

T his multicolor chili takes just thirty minutes to prepare. It's chock-full of fiber, which enhances immune function and rids the body of excess circulating hormones and carcinogens, thus lowering cancer risk. Serve it with brown rice or warmed tortillas and a green salad.

2 cups water

1 large onion, diced

1 teaspoon whole cumin seeds

1 green bell pepper, diced

6 garlic cloves, minced or pressed

1 cup crushed tomatoes or tomato sauce

2 tablespoons chili powder

1½ cups cooked or canned black beans, rinsed and drained

1½ cups cooked or canned great northern beans, rinsed and drained

1½ cups cooked or canned red beans, rinsed and drained

1½ cups bean cooking liquid, vegetable broth, or water

1. Heat ½ cup of the water in a large soup pot. Add the onion and cumin seeds and cook over high heat, stirring often, for 3 to 5 minutes, or until the onion is soft. Add a small amount of additional water if the onion begins to stick.

2. Stir in the bell pepper, garlic, and ½ cup of the remaining water. Lower the heat to medium and cook for 3 minutes, stirring occasionally. Add the tomatoes, chili powder, and remaining 1 cup of water. Cover and simmer for 5 minutes.

3. Add all of the beans and the bean cooking liquid. Cover loosely and simmer for 15 minutes.

4. Stored in a covered container in the refrigerator, leftover Three Bean Chili will keep for up to 3 days.

PER SERVING: 174 calories; 1 g fat; 0.2 g saturated fat; 5.1% calories from fat; 0 mg cholesterol; 10.8 g protein; 32.5 g carbohydrate; 3.7 g sugar; 8.3 g fiber; 395 mg sodium; 96 mg calcium; 3.9 mg iron; 16.8 mg vitamin C; 328 mcg beta-carotene; 1.3 mg vitamin E

Tomato Soup with White Beans

This version of tomato soup is heartier, chunkier, and lower in sodium than commercial brands. It also contains over 5 grams of fiber per serving. Navy, cannellini, and great northern beans all work equally well in this recipe. Serve this creamy soup with Braised Kale (page 173) and crusty bread.

1½ cups water or vegetable broth

1 small onion, diced

1 cup diced celery

½ teaspoon paprika

½ teaspoon dried basil

½ teaspoon dried thyme

¼ teaspoon ground black pepper

1 can (15 ounces) chopped tomatoes, undrained, or 1½ cups chopped fresh tomatoes

1½ cups cooked or canned white beans, rinsed and drained

½ cup bean cooking liquid, vegetable broth, or water

5 to 6 tablespoons apple juice concentrate

2 cups Basic White Sauce (page 157)

¼ to ½ teaspoon salt

1. Combine ½ cup of the water with the onion, celery, paprika, basil, thyme, and pepper in a large soup pot. Cook over medium-high heat, stirring often, for about 5 minutes, or until the onion is soft.

2. Lower the heat to medium. Stir in the remaining cup of water and the tomatoes and their liquid. Add the beans, bean cooking liquid, and apple juice concentrate. Cover and simmer for 15 minutes, stirring occasionally.

3. Add the Basic White Sauce and heat gently, stirring frequently, until the soup is very hot and steamy. Season with salt to taste.

4. Stored in a covered container in the refrigerator, leftover Tomato Soup with White Beans will keep for up to 3 days.

Note: If you prefer a smooth soup, process it in batches in a blender before adding the Basic White Sauce.

PER SERVING: 186 calories; 3.4 g fat; 0.6 g saturated fat; 16.7% calories from fat; 0 mg cholesterol; 7.8 g protein; 32.6 g carbohydrate; 8.4 g sugar; 5.4 g fiber; 556 mg sodium; 85 mg calcium; 3.6 mg iron; 8.6 mg vitamin C; 174 mcg beta-carotene; 1.2 mg vitamin E

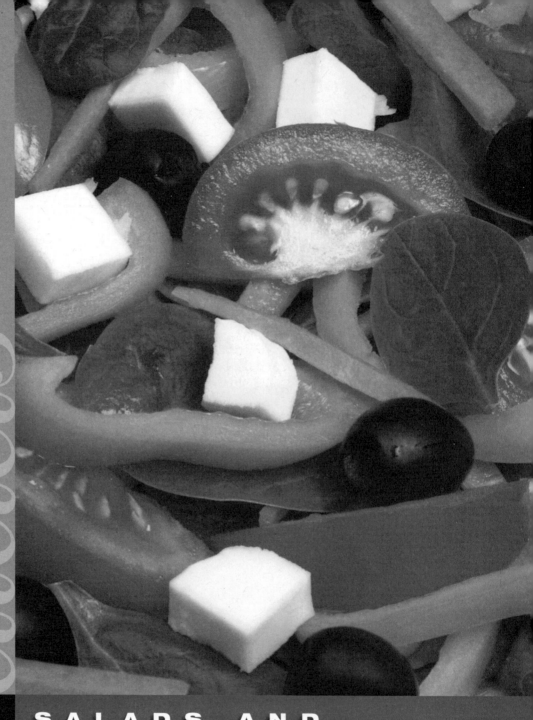

SALADS AND
SALAD DRESSINGS

Asian Fusion Salad

erved with whole-grain rolls, this vibrant salad is a meal in itself. It's so low in fat and full of antioxidants, you'll feel healthier just looking at all these cancer-fighting power foods.

1 head red leaf lettuce

1½ cups bean sprouts, rinsed and drained

1¼ cups snow peas, trimmed and cut on the diagonal into ½-inch pieces

1 large cucumber, peeled (if desired) and sliced into matchsticks

1 red bell pepper

2 carrots, cut into matchsticks

½ cup low-fat bottled salad dressing of your choice (such as sesame shiitake, lemon-tahini, or cilantro lime; optional)

1 tablespoon balsamic vinegar

1 teaspoon soy sauce

¼ teaspoon Thai chili paste or other chili sauce

1½ cups cooked or canned white beans, rinsed and drained

1. Wash the lettuce and tear it into bite-size pieces. Dry it thoroughly in a salad spinner and transfer to a large salad bowl. Add the bean sprouts, snow peas, and cucumber.

2. Cut the bell pepper into thin slices. Then cut the slices diagonally into thirds and add to the salad bowl.

3. If desired, blanch the carrots in boiling water for 3 to 4 minutes to soften. Immediately rinse them with cold water to stop the cooking process and drain well. Add the carrots to the salad bowl. Toss well. If using the optional salad dressing, add it just before serving and toss again. Make an indentation in the center of the salad.

4. Combine the vinegar, soy sauce, and chili paste in a medium bowl. Add the beans and toss until they are evenly coated. Spoon the bean mixture into the center of the salad just before serving.

PER SERVING: 94 calories; 1.8 g fat; 0.3 g saturated fat; 17.1% calories from fat; 0 mg cholesterol; 6.4 g protein; 14.8 g carbohydrate; 2.8 g sugar; 3.9 g fiber; 117 mg sodium; 64 mg calcium; 2.3 mg iron; 37.7 mg vitamin C; 2251 mcg beta-carotene; 0.8 mg vitamin E

Broccoli Salad

This colorful salad, dressed with a creamy sweet-and-sour dressing, is a delicious way to eat broccoli, one of Mother Nature's most healthful foods. Broccoli, and particularly broccoli sprouts, is an excellent source of the cancer-fighting antioxidant sulforaphane. Top this salad with the optional broccoli sprouts to pack in even more powerful cancer-fighting ingredients.

2 medium broccoli crowns with stalks

½ cup grated carrots

½ cup golden raisins

2 to 3 green onions, thinly sliced

¼ cup dried cranberries

¼ cup seasoned rice vinegar

3 tablespoons fat-free or low-fat vegan mayonnaise

1 tablespoon sugar

¼ teaspoon ground black pepper

½ to 1 cup broccoli sprouts (optional)

1. Cut the broccoli crowns into bite-size florets. Peel the broccoli stems and cut them into bite-size pieces. Transfer to a salad bowl and add the carrots, raisins, green onions, and cranberries. Toss gently.

2. Combine the vinegar, mayonnaise, sugar, and pepper in a small bowl. Pour over the broccoli mixture and toss until evenly distributed. Let stand for about 30 minutes before serving to allow the flavors to blend.

3. Top each serving with one-quarter of the broccoli sprouts if desired.

4. Stored in a covered container in the refrigerator, leftover Broccoli Salad will keep for up to 3 days.

PER SERVING: 172 calories; 3.1 g fat; 0.4 g saturated fat; 16.4% calories from fat; 0 mg cholesterol; 3.5 g protein; 36.1 g carbohydrate; 26.5 g sugar; 3.7 g fiber; 361 mg sodium; 62 mg calcium; 1.3 mg iron; 70 mg vitamin C; 1457 mcg beta-carotene; 2 mg vitamin E

Bulgur and Orange Salad

This nutritious salad contains beans, grains, vegetables, and fruit. It may be used as a side dish or served as a complete meal. It's low in fat but quite filling due to all of the wholesome fiber.

1 cup bulgur

¾ teaspoon salt

2 cups boiling water

1½ cups cooked or canned black beans, rinsed and drained

1 orange, peeled and chopped

½ red bell pepper, diced

2 green onions, thinly sliced

2 tablespoons seasoned rice vinegar

1 tablespoon orange juice concentrate

½ teaspoon ground cumin

1. Place the bulgur in a large, heatproof bowl and stir in ½ teaspoon of the salt. Add the boiling water and stir just until mixed. Cover and let stand until the bulgur is tender, about 25 minutes. Cool completely.

2. When the bulgur is cool, add the beans, orange, bell pepper, and green onions.

3. Combine the vinegar, orange juice concentrate, cumin, and remaining ¼ teaspoon of salt in a small bowl. Add to the salad and toss until evenly distributed. If time permits, chill before serving to allow the flavors to develop.

4. This salad will be even more flavorful the next day. Stored in a covered container in the refrigerator, leftover Bulgur and Orange Salad will keep for up to 3 days.

PER SERVING: 174 calories; 0.7 g fat; 0.1 g saturated fat; 3.5% calories from fat; 0 mg cholesterol; 7.5 g protein; 37 g carbohydrate; 6.9 g sugar; 8.2 g fiber; 473 mg sodium; 59 mg calcium; 2 mg iron; 33.9 mg vitamin C; 258 mcg beta-carotene; 0.3 mg vitamin E

Citrus Basil Salad

The orange in this tangy salad provides flavor and vitamin C—a potent antioxidant—which scavenges free radicals that may otherwise lead to cancer development.

1 orange, peeled and cut into chunks

1 red bell pepper, diced

1 cucumber, peeled and cut into chunks

1 cup sugar snap peas, cut in half

8 fresh basil leaves, thinly sliced

1 tablespoon seasoned rice vinegar

¼ teaspoon ground black pepper

1. Combine the orange, bell pepper, cucumber, sugar snap peas, and basil in a mixing bowl. Sprinkle with the vinegar and pepper and toss until evenly distributed.

2. Citrus Basil Salad is best served the same day it is made. If you must prepare it in advance, omit the basil, cover the salad tightly, and refrigerate it for up to 2 days. Add the basil to the salad 15 to 20 minutes prior to serving.

PER SERVING: 45 calories; 0.3 g fat; 0 g saturated fat; 5.5% calories from fat; 0 mg cholesterol; 1.7 g protein; 9.9 g carbohydrate; 6.7 g sugar; 2.5 g fiber; 62 mg sodium; 34 mg calcium; 0.8 mg iron; 87 mg vitamin C; 702 mcg beta-carotene; 0.6 mg vitamin E

Cucumber, Mango, and Spinach Salad

This salad boasts beta-carotene from the mango and lutein from the spinach, which are cousins in the carotenoid family and important antioxidants. Aside from cancer prevention and survival, lutein is recognized for its key role in eye health.

1 bag (10 ounces) **or 1 bunch fresh spinach**

1 mango, peeled and cut into bite-size pieces (see page 111)

1 large cucumber, peeled and sliced

6 green onions, thinly sliced

½ cup thinly sliced fresh basil

½ cup seasoned rice vinegar

3 tablespoons freshly squeezed lime juice

¼ teaspoon ground black pepper

1. Wash the spinach and dry it in a salad spinner. If the leaves are large, tear them into bite-size pieces. Transfer to a large salad bowl.
2. Combine the mango, cucumber, green onions, and basil in a medium bowl. Add the vinegar and lime juice and toss until evenly coated. Arrange the mango mixture on the spinach and sprinkle with the black pepper.
3. Cucumber, Mango, and Spinach Salad should be served immediately. If you must prepare the salad in advance, omit the basil and store the spinach and mango mixture separately in covered containers in the refrigerator for up to 2 days. Add the basil to the mango mixture 15 to 20 minutes before serving, and assemble and dress the salad just before serving.

PER SERVING: 45 calories; 0.3 g fat; 0 g saturated fat; 5.5% calories from fat; 0 mg cholesterol; 1.5 g protein; 10.9 g carbohydrate; 7.4 g sugar; 1.7 g fiber; 219 mg sodium; 50 mg calcium; 1.3 mg iron; 19.1 mg vitamin C; 2134 mcg beta-carotene; 1 mg vitamin E

Easy Bean Salad

T he simplicity and widespread enjoyment of this salad have made it a Cancer Project classic. Plus, it has lots of fiber to help move carcinogens and excess cholesterol and hormones out of your body to improve overall health.

1½ cups cooked or canned kidney beans, rinsed and drained

1½ cups cooked or canned pinto beans, rinsed and drained

1½ cups cooked or canned black-eyed peas, rinsed and drained

1 package (10 ounces) frozen lima beans (preferably Fordhook), thawed, 1½ cups cooked or canned lima beans, rinsed and drained, or 1½ cups cooked green soybeans (shelled edamame)

1 cup frozen corn, thawed, or cooked fresh corn, chilled

1 large red bell pepper, diced

½ medium red onion, diced

½ cup low-fat or fat-free Italian salad dressing

1 teaspoon salt

1 teaspoon ground black pepper

1. Combine all of the ingredients in a large bowl and toss gently. Serve cold or at room temperature.

2. Stored in a covered container in the refrigerator, leftover Easy Bean Salad will keep for up to 3 days.

PER SERVING: 183 calories; 3 g fat; 0.5 g saturated fat; 14.6% calories from fat; 0 mg cholesterol; 9.9 g protein; 31 g carbohydrate; 2.9 g sugar; 8 g fiber; 539 mg sodium; 43 mg calcium; 2.7 mg iron; 36.7 mg vitamin C; 311 mcg beta-carotene; 0.8 mg vitamin E

Fiesta Salad

This salad is a celebration of color and taste. It may be made in advance and keeps well for several days. It is nearly fat free, which is important when it comes to lowering cancer risk and improving survival.

4½ cups cooked or canned black beans, rinsed and drained

2 cups frozen corn, thawed

2 large tomatoes, diced

1 large green bell pepper, diced

1 large red or yellow bell pepper, diced

¾ cup minced fresh cilantro (optional)

½ cup diced red onion

3 tablespoons freshly squeezed lemon juice

2 tablespoons seasoned rice vinegar

2 tablespoons apple cider vinegar

2 teaspoons ground cumin

1 teaspoon ground coriander

2 garlic cloves, minced or pressed

½ teaspoon crushed red pepper flakes, or a pinch of cayenne

½ teaspoon salt

1. Combine the beans, corn, tomatoes, bell peppers, optional cilantro, and onion in a large bowl.
2. Whisk together the lemon juice, rice vinegar, apple cider vinegar, cumin, coriander, garlic, crushed red pepper flakes, and salt in a small bowl. Pour over the salad and toss gently until evenly distributed.
3. Stored in a covered container in the refrigerator, leftover Fiesta Salad will keep for up to 3 days.

PER SERVING: 174 calories; 1 g fat; 0.2 g saturated fat; 5.2% calories from fat; 0 mg cholesterol; 9.2 g protein; 34.9 g carbohydrate; 7 g sugar; 7.7 g fiber; 337 mg sodium; 77 mg calcium; 2.9 mg iron; 52.5 mg vitamin C; 503 mcg beta-carotene; 0.7 mg vitamin E

Hoppin' John Salad

Hoppin' John is a rice and bean dish traditionally served in the southern United States on New Year's Day to bring a year filled with luck. Eaten any time of year, however, this salad is delicious and loaded with cancer-fighting power-foods.

1½ cups cooked or canned black-eyed peas, rinsed and drained

1½ cups cooked Brown Rice (page 159)

1 tomato, diced

½ cup thinly sliced green onions

½ cup thinly sliced celery

2 tablespoons minced fresh parsley

¼ cup freshly squeezed lemon juice

1 tablespoon olive oil

1 to 2 garlic cloves, minced or pressed

¼ teaspoon salt

1. Combine the black-eyed peas, rice, tomato, green onions, celery, and parsley in a mixing bowl.

2. Whisk together the lemon juice, oil, garlic, and salt in a small bowl. Pour over the salad and toss gently until evenly distributed. If time permits, chill for 1 to 2 hours before serving to allow the flavors to blend.

3. Stored in a covered container in the refrigerator, leftover Hoppin' John Salad will keep for up to 3 days.

PER SERVING: 91 calories; 1.9 g fat; 0.3 g saturated fat; 18.5% calories from fat; 0 mg cholesterol; 3.7 g protein; 15.4 g carbohydrate; 1.3 g sugar; 3.6 g fiber; 68 mg sodium; 20 mg calcium; 1.2 mg iron; 5.4 mg vitamin C; 137 mcg beta-carotene; 0.4 mg vitamin E

Hot or Cold Beet Salad

The pigment that gives beets their rich crimson color and makes this salad so gorgeous is also a powerful cancer-fighting agent in the anthocyanin family.

3 medium beets

1½ tablespoons freshly squeezed lemon juice

1 tablespoon apple cider vinegar

1 tablespoon apple juice concentrate

1 teaspoon stone-ground mustard

½ teaspoon dried dill weed

1. Wash and peel the beets. Cut each beet in half, and each half into four wedges. To prevent staining your countertop, place a dark-colored towel or paper towels under your cutting board.

2. Steam the beets over boiling water until tender when pierced with a fork, 15 to 20 minutes.

3. Combine the lemon juice, vinegar, apple juice concentrate, mustard, and dill weed in a serving bowl. Add beets and toss to mix. Serve hot or cold.

4. Stored in a covered container in the refrigerator, leftover Hot or Cold Beet Salad will keep for up to 3 days.

PER SERVING: 36 calories; 0.2 g fat; 0 g saturated fat; 4.9% calories from fat; 0 mg cholesterol; 1 g protein; 8.4 g carbohydrate; 7 g sugar; 1.1 g fiber; 61 mg sodium; 15 mg calcium; 0.6 mg iron; 4 mg vitamin C; 21 mcg beta-carotene; 0.1 mg vitamin E

Lentil and Bulgur Salad

The garlic in this tangy salad contains a potent cancer-fighter called allicin, which has been shown to help the body eliminate carcinogens and slow the growth of cancer cells. Serve this salad with wedges of fresh pita bread for a very satisfying meal.

4½ cups water

1 cup dried brown or green lentils

1 cup bulgur

1 cucumber, peeled, seeded, and diced

1 ripe tomato, diced

3 green onions, thinly sliced

¼ cup freshly squeezed lemon juice

3 garlic cloves, minced or pressed

1 teaspoon salt

1. Bring 2½ cups of the water to a boil in a medium saucepan. Add the lentils, lower the heat, cover, and simmer for 25 to 30 minutes, or until tender. Check occasionally and add a small amount of extra water, if necessary, so the lentils don't cook dry. Remove from the heat and let cool.

2. Place the remaining 2 cups of water in a small saucepan and bring to a boil. Add the bulgur, stir, remove from the heat, and cover. Let stand for about 25 minutes, until the bulgur is tender and all of the water has been absorbed. Let cool.

3. When the lentils and bulgur have cooled, combine them in a large bowl with the cucumber, tomato, green onions, lemon juice, garlic, and salt. Toss until evenly combined.

4. The flavors of this salad are best when it is served at room temperature. Leftover Lentil and Bulgur Salad will keep in a covered container in the refrigerator for up to 3 days.

PER SERVING: 162 calories; 2.3 g fat; 0.3 g saturated fat; 12.6% calories from fat; 0 mg cholesterol; 8.6 g protein; 29 g carbohydrate; 1.6 g sugar; 7.6 g fiber; 304 mg sodium; 32 mg calcium; 2.9 mg iron; 7.1 mg vitamin C; 115 mcg beta-carotene; 0.5 mg vitamin E

Potato Salad

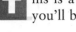

This is a low-fat version of the traditional summertime favorite. You won't miss the fat and you'll be healthier for it! You can use any variety of potato that you like.

2 medium potatoes, peeled (if desired) **and cut into ½-inch cubes** (about 2½ cups)

½ cup diced sweet onion

½ cup diced celery

½ small red bell pepper, finely diced

¼ cup minced fresh parsley

1 teaspoon dried dill weed

¼ cup fat-free or low-fat vegan mayonnaise

1 tablespoon seasoned rice vinegar

1½ teaspoons mustard

⅛ teaspoon salt

⅛ teaspoon ground black pepper

1. Steam the potatoes until just barely tender when pierced with a knife, about 10 minutes. Do not overcook. Transfer to a large bowl and add the onion, celery, bell pepper, parsley, and dill weed.

2. In a separate bowl, combine the mayonnaise, vinegar, mustard, salt, and pepper. Mix well. Add to the potato mixture and toss gently until evenly distributed. Chill thoroughly before serving.

3. Stored in a covered container in the refrigerator, leftover Potato Salad will keep for up to 3 days.

PER SERVING: 135 calories; 3.8 g fat; 0.5 g saturated fat; 25.1% calories from fat; 0 mg cholesterol; 2.9 g protein; 23.7 g carbohydrate; 4.7 g sugar; 3.4 g fiber; 289 mg sodium; 46 mg calcium; 2.3 mg iron; 36.4 mg vitamin C; 394 mcg beta-carotene; 1.1 mg vitamin E

Salad of Spicy Greens with Fruit and Pine Nuts

This colorful salad is a delightful blend of flavors. Spicy greens are available at supermarkets, natural food stores, and farmers' markets. Examples are arugula, mizuna, watercress, radicchio, red mustard, or Belgian endive. You can also use a prewashed salad mix that contains these greens.

6 cups mixed spicy greens

1 ripe pear, diced

1 tangerine, seeded and sectioned

2 tablespoons balsamic vinegar

2 tablespoons apple juice concentrate

¼ teaspoon salt

1 to 2 tablespoons raw pine nuts

¼ teaspoon ground black pepper

1. Wash the greens and pat dry or dry in a salad spinner. Tear any large leaves into bite-size pieces. Place in a bowl and add the pear and tangerine.

2. To make the dressing, combine the vinegar, apple juice concentrate, and salt in a jar. Just before serving, shake the dressing and pour it over the salad. Toss gently to mix. Divide the salad among individual serving plates and sprinkle with the pine nuts and pepper.

3. Salad of Spicy Greens with Fruit and Pine Nuts is best served immediately. If you need to make the salad in advance, store the greens and fruit separately in covered containers in the refrigerator for up to 3 days. Toss with the dressing and garnish with the pine nuts and pepper just before serving.

PER SERVING: 48 calories; 1.1 g fat; 0.1 g saturated fat; 21.2% calories from fat; 0 mg cholesterol; 1.1 g protein; 9.7 g carbohydrate; 6.3 g sugar; 1.6 g fiber; 110 mg sodium; 33 mg calcium; 0.4 mg iron; 12.6 mg vitamin C; 442 mcg beta-carotene; 0.6 mg vitamin E

Southwest Bean Salad

This salad is a tasty way to use leftover cooked grains. You'll find vegetarian chili beans in most supermarkets and natural food stores. This recipe contains about 7 grams of fiber per serving.

1 to 2 cups cooked Brown Rice (page 159), **Bulgur** (page 162), **millet, quinoa,** or **other whole grain**

1½ cups cooked or canned chili beans, rinsed and drained

1 cup fresh or frozen corn, thawed

1 cup diced sweet onion

1 cup diced celery

1 small green or red bell pepper, diced

½ cup minced fresh cilantro

1 tablespoon seasoned rice vinegar

2 garlic cloves, minced or pressed

½ teaspoon salt

Dash of hot sauce

1. Combine all of the ingredients in a bowl and toss gently to mix.
2. Let stand at room temperature for about 30 minutes before serving to allow the flavors to develop.
3. Stored in a covered container in the refrigerator, leftover Southwest Bean Salad will keep for up to 3 days.

PER SERVING: 175 calories; 1.2 g fat; 0.2 g saturated fat; 6% calories from fat; 0 mg cholesterol; 6.8 g protein; 37 g carbohydrate; 7.1 g sugar; 6.6 g fiber; 895 mg sodium; 55 mg calcium; 1.9 mg iron; 24.5 mg vitamin C; 310 mcg beta-carotene; 0.8 mg vitamin E

Spinach Salad with Citrus Fruit

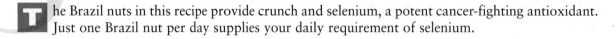

he Brazil nuts in this recipe provide crunch and selenium, a potent cancer-fighting antioxidant. Just one Brazil nut per day supplies your daily requirement of selenium.

1 bag (10 ounces) **spinach, chopped**

1 can (10 ounces) **mandarin or clementine oranges or grapefruit sections, rinsed and drained, or 1⅓ cups fresh clementine orange or grapefruit sections**

1 cup berries or grapes, or 10 strawberries, sliced

¼ cup fat-free raspberry vinaigrette

1 tablespoon raw sunflower seeds

1 tablespoon chopped Brazil nuts

1. Combine all of the ingredients in a bowl and toss gently to mix.
2. Serve immediately.

PER SERVING: 62 calories; 2 g fat; 0.3 g saturated fat; 29.4% calories from fat; 0 mg cholesterol; 2.3 g protein; 10.1 g carbohydrate; 5.4 g sugar; 2.4 g fiber; 61 mg sodium; 59 mg calcium; 1.7 mg iron; 36.7 mg vitamin C; 2746 mcg beta-carotene; 1.7 mg vitamin E

Spinach Salad with Orange, Radicchio, and Sesame

Spinach and radicchio, garnished with tangy citrus and flavorful sesame seeds, make a colorful salad. Sesame seeds are a great source of highly absorbable calcium and vitamin E, known for its antioxidant activity.

2 tablespoons apple juice concentrate

1 tablespoon orange juice concentrate

1 tablespoon balsamic vinegar

½ teaspoon potato flour

¼ teaspoon salt

1 bag (10 ounces) **spinach**

2 cups loosely packed radicchio leaves

1 orange, peeled, seeded, separated into sections, and cut into bite-size pieces

2 to 3 tablespoons unhulled raw sesame seeds

1. To make the dressing, combine the apple juice concentrate, orange juice concentrate, vinegar, flour, and salt in a small bowl. Mix well and set aside.

2. Wash the spinach and radicchio and pat dry or dry in a salad spinner. If the leaves are large, tear them into bite-size pieces. Place in a salad bowl and add the orange pieces.

3. Toast the sesame seeds for about 2 to 3 minutes in a heavy skillet over medium-high heat, stirring constantly, until they become fragrant and begin to pop. Remove from the skillet and let cool.

4. Just before serving, add the dressing to the spinach mixture and toss until evenly distributed. Sprinkle with the sesame seeds and serve immediately.

PER SERVING: 41 calories; 1.3 g fat; 0.2 g saturated fat; 27.5% calories from fat; 0 mg cholesterol; 1.6 g protein; 7 g carbohydrate; 4.2 g sugar; 1.5 g fiber; 101 mg sodium; 62 mg calcium; 1.3 mg iron; 21.1 mg vitamin C; 1703 mcg beta-carotene; 0.9 mg vitamin E

Tomato, Cucumber, and Basil Salad

This tomato-based salad is rich in lycopene, a powerful carotenoid that has proven its importance in prostate cancer prevention and survival.

4 tomatoes, quartered and sliced

½ large cucumber, peeled, quartered, and sliced

½ cup fresh basil leaves

3 to 4 tablespoons balsamic vinegar

¼ teaspoon ground black pepper

1. Arrange the tomatoes and cucumber in a shallow bowl.
2. Scatter the basil leaves on top and sprinkle with the vinegar and pepper.
3. Tomato, Cucumber, and Basil Salad is best served at room temperature shortly after it has been made.

PER SERVING: 20 calories; 0.2 g fat; 0 g saturated fat; 10.4% calories from fat; 0 mg cholesterol; 1 g protein; 4.3 g carbohydrate; 2.5 g sugar; 1.3 g fiber; 5 mg sodium; 17 mg calcium; 0.4 mg iron; 11.8 mg vitamin C; 487 mcg beta-carotene; 0.5 mg vitamin E; 2110 mcg lycopene

Raspberry Salad Dressing

his dressing is virtually fat free and is delicious on Spinach Salad with Citrus Fruit (page 148).

2 cups fresh or frozen raspberries, thawed and drained

1 to 2 tablespoons balsamic vinegar

1 tablespoon finely chopped fresh herbs, such as thyme or rosemary (optional)

2 teaspoons Dijon mustard or grainy mustard

1 to 2 teaspoons maple syrup

¼ teaspoon salt

¼ teaspoon ground black pepper

1. Purée the raspberries in a food processor or blender. Transfer to a bowl and whisk in all of the remaining ingredients, starting with 1 tablespoon of the vinegar and adding more after tasting. Adjust the flavor by adding more maple syrup, salt, or pepper to taste.

2. Stored in a covered container in the refrigerator, leftover Raspberry Salad Dressing will keep for up to 3 days.

PER SERVING: 22 calories; 0.3 g fat; 0 g saturated fat; 11.8% calories from fat; 0 mg cholesterol; 0.5 g protein; 4.7 g carbohydrate; 2.2 g sugar; 2.1 g fiber; 179 mg sodium; 10 mg calcium; 0.3 mg iron; 8.2 mg vitamin C; 10 mcg beta-carotene; 0.3 mg vitamin E

Piquant Dressing

T his dressing has a Mexican flavor. It can be as spicy as the salsa you use to make it.

¼ cup seasoned rice vinegar

¼ cup salsa

1 garlic clove, pressed

1. Whisk together all of the ingredients in a small bowl.
2. Stored in a covered container in the refrigerator, Piquant Dressing will keep for up to 1 week.

PER SERVING: 13 calories; 0 g fat; 0 g saturated fat; 1% calories from fat; 0 mg cholesterol; 0.2 g protein; 3.1 g carbohydrate; 2.6 g sugar; 0.1 g fiber; 167 mg sodium; 3 mg calcium; 0.1 mg iron; 0.3 mg vitamin C; 14 mcg beta-carotene; 0.1 mg vitamin E

Balsamic Vinaigrette

T he mellow flavor of balsamic vinegar is delicious on any green salad.

2 tablespoons balsamic vinegar

2 tablespoons seasoned rice vinegar

1 tablespoon ketchup

1 teaspoon stone-ground mustard

1 garlic clove, pressed

1. Whisk together all of the ingredients in a small bowl.
2. Stored in a covered container in the refrigerator, Balsamic Vinaigrette will keep for up to 2 weeks.

PER SERVING: 17 calories; 0.1 g fat; 0 g saturated fat; 3% calories from fat; 0 mg cholesterol; 0.2 g protein; 3.8 g carbohydrate; 3.3 g sugar; 0.1 g fiber; 175 mg sodium; 4 mg calcium; 0.1 mg iron; 0.8 mg vitamin C; 22 mcg beta-carotene; 0.1 mg vitamin E

Creamy Dill Dressing

 This rich-tasting, creamy dressing has no added oil. Its creaminess comes from tofu.

1 package (12.3 ounces) firm silken tofu

2 tablespoons freshly squeezed lemon juice

3 tablespoons seasoned rice vinegar

1 tablespoon apple cider vinegar

1 teaspoon garlic powder

½ teaspoon dried dill weed

¼ teaspoon salt

1. Combine all of the ingredients in a food processor or blender and process for 1 to 2 minutes, until completely smooth.
2. Stored in a covered container in the refrigerator, Creamy Dill Dressing will keep for up to 1 week.

PER SERVING: 12 calories; 0.4 g fat; 0.1 g saturated fat; 28.8% calories from fat; 0 mg cholesterol; 1 g protein; 1.2 g carbohydrate; 0.9 g sugar; 0 g fiber; 60 mg sodium; 5 mg calcium; 0.2 mg iron; 0.4 mg vitamin C; 1 mcg beta-carotene; 0 mg vitamin E

Sauces

SAUCES AND GRAVIES

Chunky Ratatouille Sauce

This sauce is loaded with vegetables, which add fiber and a variety of important cancer fighters. It's delicious when served over pasta shells, brown rice, or your favorite whole grain.

1 large eggplant, unpeeled, cut into 1-inch chunks

½ cup red wine or vegetable broth

2 small onions, diced

2 celery stalks, diced

6 garlic cloves, minced

¼ to ½ cup water

8 ounces cremini mushrooms, sliced

1 can (15 ounces) fire-roasted tomatoes

1 teaspoon Italian seasoning

½ teaspoon dried thyme

½ teaspoon ground black pepper

1. Soak the eggplant chunks in salted water for 10 minutes. Drain, rinse, and drain again.

2. Heat ¼ cup of the wine in a nonstick skillet. Add the onions, celery, and garlic, cover, and cook over medium heat for 10 to 15 minutes, or until soft, stirring occasionally and adding more wine if the vegetables start to stick.

3. When the onions and celery are soft, add the eggplant and ¼ cup of the water. Simmer for 8 to 10 minutes, stirring occasionally, until the eggplant is soft. Add more water as needed to keep the mixture from drying out.

4. Stir in the mushrooms, tomatoes, Italian seasoning, thyme, pepper, and the remaining ¼ cup of wine and simmer for 5 minutes.

5. Stored in a covered container in the refrigerator, leftover Chunky Ratatouille Sauce will keep for up to 4 days.

PER SERVING: 88 calories; 0.6 g fat; 0.1 g saturated fat; 5.7% calories from fat; 0 mg cholesterol; 2.7 g protein; 17.6 g total carbohydrate; 7.4 g sugar; 4.6 g fiber; 106 mg sodium; 52 mg calcium; 1.9 mg iron; 11.7 mg vitamin C; 124 mcg beta-carotene; 1 mg vitamin E

Mushroom Gravy

This gravy is delicious over Mashed Grains and Cauliflower (page 168), but enjoy it with any dish that can handle a scrumptious, nutritious gravy.

¼ cup water

12 ounces mushrooms (button, cremini, or your favorite kind), **sliced**

1½ cups vegetable broth

¼ cup flour (any kind)

1 to 2 tablespoons soy sauce (optional)

1 teaspoon Italian seasoning

¼ teaspoon salt

¼ teaspoon ground black pepper

1. Heat the water in a nonstick skillet. Add the mushrooms and cook and stir until soft.

2. Combine 1 cup of the broth and all of the flour in a jar with a tight-fitting lid and shake until smooth.

3. Add the remaining ½ cup of the broth, the optional soy sauce, the Italian seasoning, and about half of the flour mixture to the mushrooms. Simmer for 3 to 5 minutes, stirring often.

4. Stir in the remaining flour mixture and cook and stir until thickened. Season with salt and pepper to taste. Serve warm, as soon as possible.

5. Stored in a covered container in the refrigerator, leftover Mushroom Gravy will keep for up to 3 days.

PER SERVING: 50 calories; 0.4 g fat; 0.1 g saturated fat; 6.8% calories from fat; 0 mg cholesterol; 2.2 g protein; 10.3 g carbohydrate; 1.1 g sugar; 1.7 g fiber; 524 mg sodium; 13 mg calcium; 1.6 mg iron; 2.8 mg vitamin C; 233 mcg beta-carotene; 0.1 mg vitamin E; 277 mcg lycopene

Simple Marinara

It doesn't get easier than this! Tomatoes, especially cooked tomatoes, are a rich source of lycopene, which has been proven to greatly reduce prostate cancer risk and even increase survival. Serve this sauce over pasta or polenta.

1 can (28 ounces) **tomato sauce**, or 3½ cups crushed tomatoes

6 fresh basil leaves, thinly sliced

1 teaspoon dried oregano

2 garlic cloves, minced or pressed

1. Combine all of the ingredients in a medium saucepan. Cook and stir over low heat for about 10 minutes, until bubbly.

2. Stored in a covered container, leftover Simple Marinara will keep for up to 3 days in the refrigerator or up to 1 month in the freezer.

PER SERVING: 67 calories; 0.5 g fat; 0.1 g saturated fat; 6.9% calories from fat; 0 mg cholesterol; 2.8 g protein; 15.3 g carbohydrate; 8.5 g sugar; 3.1 g fiber; 1040 mg sodium; 34 mg calcium; 2.2 mg iron; 14.6 mg vitamin C; 449 mcg beta-carotene; 4.2 mg vitamin E; 30069 mcg lycopene

Simple Brown Gravy

This gravy is low in fat and takes just minutes to prepare. Serve it with No-Meat Loaf (page 195), Garlic Mashed Potatoes (page 177), and green beans for a wonderful, traditional meal.

1½ cups water

2 tablespoons soy sauce

2 tablespoons raw cashews

4 teaspoons potato flour

1 tablespoon onion powder

½ teaspoon garlic powder

½ teaspoon dried thyme

⅛ teaspoon ground black pepper

1. Combine all of the ingredients in a blender and process until completely smooth. Transfer to a saucepan and simmer, stirring constantly, until thickened.

2. Stored in a covered container in the refrigerator, leftover Simple Brown Gravy will keep for up to 2 days.

PER SERVING: 31 calories; 1.3 g fat; 0.2 g saturated fat; 37.7% calories from fat; 0 mg cholesterol; 1.1 g protein; 4.3 g carbohydrate; 0.7 g sugar; 0.4 g fiber; 307 mg sodium; 11 mg calcium; 0.4 mg iron; 0.4 mg vitamin C; 2 mcg beta-carotene; 0 mg vitamin E

Basic White Sauce

This creamy sauce is low in fat and cholesterol free. Use it for making creamed soups, sauces, and gravies. Be sure to continue blending the ingredients until they are completely smooth; this can take up to two minutes on the highest speed. The first few times you make this sauce, give it a taste test to make certain it is smooth and creamy before proceeding.

2⅓ cups water

⅓ cup millet

¼ cup raw cashews

½ teaspoon salt

1. Combine 1⅓ cups of the water with the millet in a saucepan. Bring to a simmer. Cover and cook for about 55 minutes, stirring occasionally, until the millet is tender and all of the water has been absorbed.

2. Transfer the millet to a blender. Add the remaining cup of water and all of the cashews and salt. Blend for 1 to 2 minutes, until completely smooth.

3. Stored in a covered container in the refrigerator, leftover Basic White Sauce will keep for up to 2 days.

PER SERVING: 55 calories; 2.3 g fat; 0.4 g saturated fat; 37.3% calories from fat; 0 mg cholesterol; 1.6 g protein; 7.3 g carbohydrate; 0.3 g sugar; 0.9 g fiber; 149 mg sodium; 3 mg calcium; 0.5 mg iron; 0 mg vitamin C; 2 mcg beta-carotene; 0 mg vitamin E

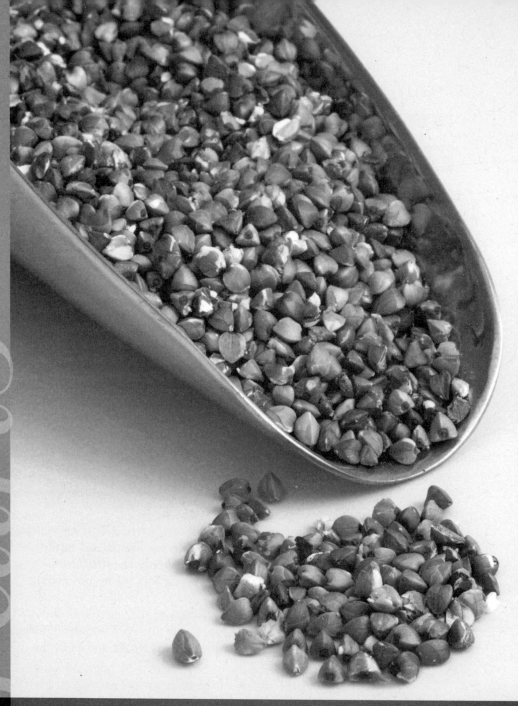

Grains

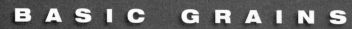

BASIC GRAINS

Brown Rice

Brown rice is higher in fiber and nutrients than white rice and has a wonderful nutty taste. There are many different varieties of brown rice, each with a slightly different flavor and texture. The long-grain varieties, which tend to be light and fluffy, are excellent for making a pilaf. The short-grain varieties are denser and chewier, making them good additions to burgers and loaves. In recent years a number of aromatic varieties, which are especially fragrant and flavorful, have been introduced. Two favorites are brown basmati and jasmine. These are sold in many supermarkets as well as in natural food stores and specialty shops.

1 cup brown rice, rinsed and drained

2 cups boiling water or vegetable broth

½ teaspoon salt

1. Place the rice in a medium saucepan over medium heat and stir constantly until it is dry and fragrant. Remove from the heat and allow the pan to cool slightly.

2. Slowly add the boiling water and salt. Cover and cook over low heat for about 50 minutes, until tender.

3. Stored in a covered container in the refrigerator, Brown Rice will keep for up to 3 days.

PER SERVING: 115 calories; 0.9 g fat; 0.2 g saturated fat; 7.3% calories from fat; 0 mg cholesterol; 2.7 g protein; 23.7 g carbohydrate; 0.4 g sugar; 3.4 g fiber; 202 mg sodium; 10 mg calcium; 0.4 mg iron; 0 mg vitamin C; 0 mcg beta-carotene; 0 mg vitamin E

Basic Polenta

P olenta is a delicious whole-grain food made from yellow corn grits. It pairs well with many different flavors, although it is typically associated with northern Italian cuisine. Corn grits come in fine, medium, or coarse grinds. Any type of corn grits can be used in this recipe, but the cooking time will increase slightly for coarser grinds.

4 cups water or vegetable broth

¼ teaspoon salt

1 cup yellow corn grits (polenta)

2 tablespoons nutritional yeast flakes

2 tablespoons chopped roasted garlic (optional; see sidebar)

2 tablespoons finely chopped fresh herbs (such as parsley, thyme, sage, or rosemary; optional)

1. Combine the water and salt in a 4-quart or larger saucepan and bring to a boil. Add the corn grits slowly while whisking continuously. Whisk for 1 to 2 minutes to prevent the mixture from lumping. Lower the heat, cover, and cook on the lowest setting for about 40 minutes, stirring often.

2. Use caution when removing the lid and stirring, as hot polenta can bubble up and splatter. If the polenta gets too thick, add a little more water or broth. If the liquid is heated before it is added, the polenta will cook faster (cold liquids will lower the polenta's temperature and extend the cooking time). The polenta is ready when it is smooth and thick and the grains are tender.

3. Toward the end of the cooking time, whisk in the nutritional yeast and optional garlic and herbs. Add more salt if needed.

4. Serve soft-style, straight from the saucepan. Alternatively, spread the polenta in a 9 x 13-inch baking dish or sheet pan and allow it to cool. Cooled polenta can be sliced, brushed with a little olive oil, and then baked in the oven or placed under a broiler until crispy.

5. Stored in a covered container in the refrigerator, leftover Basic Polenta will keep for up to 4 days. When reheating soft-style polenta, thin it by whisking in a little vegetable broth or water.

PER SERVING: 164 calories; 1 g fat; 0.1 g saturated fat; 5.2% calories from fat; 0 mg cholesterol; 5.2 g protein; 33.6 g carbohydrate; 0.7 g sugar; 2.7 g fiber; 160 mg sodium; 14 mg calcium; 2.1 mg iron; 2.5 mg vitamin C; 133 mcg beta-carotene; 0.1 mg vitamin E

How to Roast Garlic

Preheat the oven to 350 degrees F. Place 8 unpeeled cloves of garlic in a small, shallow baking dish. Using your hands, coat the cloves with 2 teaspoons of olive oil. Add 1 to 2 teaspoons of water or vegetable broth and sprinkle with a little salt. Cover with a lid or foil and roast in the oven for about 30 minutes. When ready, the garlic should be very soft and golden brown. Squeeze the pulp out of the skins to use.

Brown Rice and Barley

B oth brown rice and barley are good sources of protective soluble fiber, and the textures of the two grains make them a most pleasing combination. Enjoy this recipe as a warm breakfast cereal topped with fresh fruit. Alternatively, serve it as a side dish or add it to soups and salads.

½ cup brown rice

½ cup pearl barley
(not quick-cooking)

2 cups boiling water or
vegetable broth

½ teaspoon salt

1. Combine the rice and barley in a strainer. Rinse under cold water and drain. Transfer to a saucepan and place over medium heat. Stir constantly until the grains are dry and have a nutty fragrance. Remove from the heat and allow the pan to cool slightly.

2. Stir in the boiling water and salt. Bring to a very low simmer, cover, and cook over low heat for about 50 minutes, until the grains are tender and all of the water has been absorbed.

3. Stored in a covered container in the refrigerator, leftover Brown Rice and Barley will keep for up to 3 days.

PER SERVING: 131 calories; 0.7 g fat; 0.1 g saturated fat; 4.9% calories from fat; 0 mg cholesterol; 3.4 g protein; 28 g carbohydrate; 0.5 g sugar; 5 g fiber; 202 mg sodium; 12 mg calcium; 0.7 mg iron; 0 mg vitamin C; 3 mcg beta-carotene; 0 mg vitamin E

Bulgur

Bulgur, which is similar to cracked wheat, has a pleasant, nutty flavor. It cooks quickly and is very versatile. Serve it as a hot breakfast cereal, pilaf, or side dish, or use it as an ingredient in soups or salads. Bulgur can be simmered for a soft texture, or it can be soaked in boiling water when a firmer, fluffier texture is desired.

1 cup bulgur

½ teaspoon salt

2 cups boiling water

1. For the simmer method, combine the bulgur and salt in a saucepan. Then stir in the boiling water. Bring to a simmer, cover, and cook over low heat until the bulgur is tender and all of the water has been absorbed, about 15 minutes.

2. For the soaking method, combine the bulgur and salt in a bowl. Then stir in the boiling water. Cover and let stand about 25 minutes, or until the bulgur is tender. Drain off any excess water.

3. Stored in a covered container in the refrigerator, leftover Bulgur will keep for up to 3 days.

PER SERVING: 80 calories; 0.3 g fat; 0.1 g saturated fat; 3.5% calories from fat; 0 mg cholesterol; 2.9 g protein; 17.7 g carbohydrate; 0.2 g sugar; 4.3 g fiber; 202 mg sodium; 10 mg calcium; 0.6 mg iron; 0 mg vitamin C; 1 mcg beta-carotene; 0 mg vitamin E

Couscous

ouscous is a tiny pasta that is cooked and served like a grain. It is quick to prepare and can be used in a wide array of dishes including pilafs, salads, and soups. Whole wheat couscous is the most nutritious. Look for it at natural food stores and larger supermarkets, or you can order it from online retailers.

1½ cups boiling water

1 cup couscous

½ teaspoon salt

1. Combine the boiling water, couscous, and salt in a saucepan or heatproof bowl. Remove from the heat, cover, and let stand for 10 to 15 minutes. Fluff with a fork before serving.

2. Stored in a covered container in the refrigerator, leftover Couscous will keep for up to 3 days.

PER SERVING: 113 calories; 0.2 g fat; 0 g saturated fat; 1.5% calories from fat; 0 mg cholesterol; 3.8 g protein; 23.2 g carbohydrate; 0.6 g sugar; 1.5 g fiber; 201 mg sodium; 9 mg calcium; 0.3 mg iron; 0 mg vitamin C; 1 mcg beta-carotene; 0 mg vitamin E

How to Toast Grains

Toasting grains before cooking them adds great flavor without any additional ingredients. Any grain—such as brown rice, couscous, millet, or quinoa—can be toasted before it is cooked. Simply place the grain in a dry saucepan over medium-high heat and cook, stirring constantly, until the grain darkens slightly, about 5 minutes. Remove from the heat and add the standard amount of water called for to cook the particular grain you are using. (See table 4, page 15, for amounts of water and cooking times for a variety of grains.) Bring to a boil, lower the heat, and cook until all of the water has been absorbed (the amount of time will vary depending on the grain used).

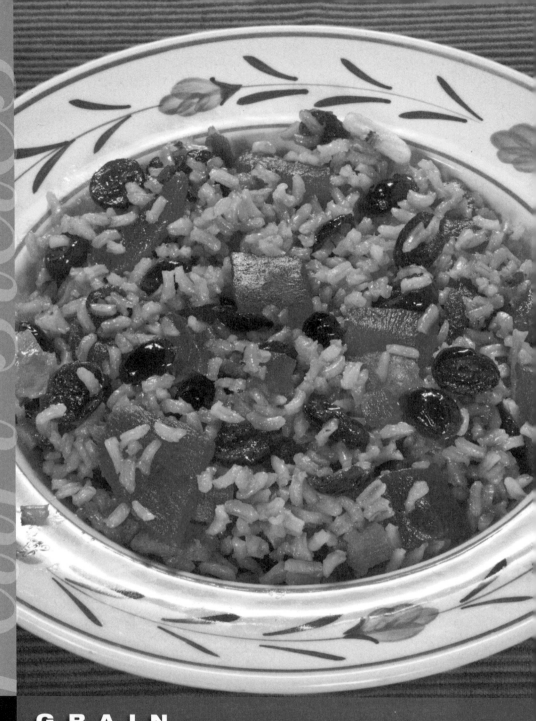

GRAIN
SIDE DISHES

Brown Rice Pilaf

This richly flavored pilaf may be served as a side dish or used as a stuffing. Brown rice is a rich source of fiber, vitamins, and minerals. Most of the nutrients available in brown rice come from the bran. When rice is processed and the bran is removed, it becomes white rice, which is essentially devoid of nutritional value and health-promoting properties.

¼ cup water

8 ounces mushrooms, diced (about 2½ cups)

1 onion, diced

2 garlic cloves, minced or pressed

½ teaspoon dried thyme

½ cup dry white wine or vegetable broth

1 cup long-grain brown rice (preferably basmati or jasmine)

2 to 3 cups boiling water or vegetable broth

½ teaspoon salt

¼ teaspoon ground black pepper

1. Heat the ¼ cup of water in a large saucepan. Add the mushrooms, onion, and garlic. Cook and stir over medium heat for 5 to 10 minutes, until the mushrooms and onion are soft.

2. Add the thyme and cook and stir for 2 to 3 minutes. Add 2 tablespoons of the wine and mix in well.

3. Stir in the rice and 2 cups of the boiling water. Add the remaining wine and the salt and pepper. Stir to mix well. Cover and cook over low heat for about 60 minutes, until the rice is tender and all of the water has been absorbed. Check the saucepan occasionally to make sure the rice doesn't cook dry, and add a small amount of the remaining water as needed to prevent sticking.

4. Stored in a covered container in the refrigerator, leftover Brown Rice Pilaf will keep for up to 3 days.

PER SERVING: 216 calories; 1.6 g fat; 0.3 g saturated fat; 6.8% calories from fat; 0 mg cholesterol; 5.3 g protein; 40.9 g carbohydrate; 2 g sugar; 6.4 g fiber; 306 mg sodium; 32 mg calcium; 1.7 mg iron; 3.3 mg vitamin C; 3 mcg beta-carotene; 0.1 mg vitamin E

Brown Rice with Black Beans

ofrito, the main flavor component of this dish, contains ingredients that have many antioxidants and cancer-fighting compounds.

Sofrito

¼ cup water

1 red bell pepper, diced

1 green bell pepper, diced

½ onion, diced

3 garlic cloves, minced or pressed

1 teaspoon ground turmeric

1 teaspoon ground cumin

½ teaspoon salt

Rice and Black Beans

3 cups water

2 cups vegetable broth

4 cups medium-grain brown rice

3 cups cooked or canned black beans, rinsed and drained

2 tablespoons chopped fresh cilantro (optional)

1. To make the sofrito, heat the water in a medium saucepan. Add the bell peppers, onion, and garlic and cook and stir for 5 minutes. If the mixture sticks, add a little more water. Stir in the turmeric, cumin, and salt. Cook on medium heat for 5 minutes longer.

2. To make the rice, bring the water and broth to a boil in a large saucepan. Add the rice, lower the heat, cover, and cook for 35 minutes, or until the rice is tender and all of the liquid has been absorbed.

3. Add the beans and sofrito mixture to the rice and cook over low heat, stirring frequently, for 10 minutes. Stir in the optional cilantro and serve.

4. Stored in a covered container in the refrigerator, leftover Brown Rice with Black Beans will keep for up to 3 days.

PER SERVING: 446 calories; 3.3 g fat; 0.7 g saturated fat; 6.7% calories from fat; 0 mg cholesterol; 14.2 g protein; 90.4 g carbohydrate; 5.3 g sugar; 16.5 g fiber; 415 mg sodium; 59 mg calcium; 3.1 mg iron; 36 mg vitamin C; 492 mcg beta-carotene; 0.5 mg vitamin E

Chinese Fried Bulgur

Mung bean sprouts are a rich source of protein and vitamins A, B, C, and E. In just one cup of mung bean sprouts there are 3 grams of protein and 0 grams of fat. Since sprouts can sometimes harbor bacteria, it is important to always rinse them thoroughly before using. Serve this colorful and crunchy bulgur pilaf with Pan-Seared Portobello Mushrooms (page 206). For a variation, substitute two and a half cups of cooked brown rice for the bulgur.

1 cup bulgur

½ teaspoon salt

2 cups boiling water

¼ cup vegetable broth or water

½ cup thinly sliced celery

½ cup diced red bell pepper

3 green onions, thinly sliced

2 garlic cloves, minced or pressed

1 teaspoon peeled and minced fresh ginger

2 cups coarsely chopped fresh bean sprouts

1 cup canned sliced water chestnuts, drained

3 to 4 tablespoons soy sauce

¼ teaspoon ground black pepper

1. Place the bulgur and salt in a saucepan or heatproof bowl. Add the boiling water and stir just until mixed. Cover and let stand for about 25 minutes, until the bulgur is tender and all of the water has been absorbed. The bulgur should be tender but not mushy. Fluff with a fork, cover, and set aside.

2. Heat the vegetable broth in a nonstick skillet over medium heat. Add the celery, bell pepper, green onions, garlic, and ginger. Cook and stir for about 3 minutes, until the vegetables just begin to soften. Add more broth or water as needed to prevent sticking.

3. Stir in the bulgur, 1 cup at a time, mixing well after each addition.

4. Add the bean sprouts and water chestnuts and sprinkle with the soy sauce and black pepper. Toss gently to mix. Cook over medium heat for about 3 minutes, turning with a spatula, until heated through. Serve immediately.

5. Stored in a covered container in the refrigerator, leftover Chinese Fried Bulgur will keep for up to 3 days.

PER SERVING: 200 calories; 2.9 g fat; 0.4 g saturated fat; 13.1% calories from fat; 0 mg cholesterol; 10.4 g protein; 38.8 g carbohydrate; 3.5 g sugar; 8.5 g fiber; 1072 mg sodium; 64 mg calcium; 2.3 mg iron; 43 mg vitamin C; 551 mcg beta-carotene; 0.6 mg vitamin E

Mashed Grains and Cauliflower

This recipe is a sneaky way to enjoy cauliflower, a star vegetable in the cruciferous family. Cruciferous vegetables contain unique cancer-fighting phytochemicals called isothiocyanates. If you like, top this dish with Mushroom Gravy (page 156).

¼ cup vegetable broth or water

1 cup diced onion

2 cups millet or quinoa, rinsed and drained, couscous, or other favorite grain

4 cups chopped cauliflower

½ teaspoon sea salt

Water for cooking 2 cups of selected grain (see table 4, page 15)

1. Heat 2 tablespoons of the broth in a large saucepan. Add the onion and cook and stir for 3 minutes, adding more broth as needed to prevent sticking.

2. Add the grain and cook and stir for 5 minutes. Add the cauliflower, salt, and water. Cover and cook according to the time listed in table 4 (page 15), or until the grain has absorbed all of the water.

3. When the grain is done, mash the mixture with a potato masher. Add a little additional water or vegetable broth, if necessary, in order to obtain a smooth consistency.

4. Stored in a covered container in the refrigerator, leftover Mashed Grains and Cauliflower will keep for up to 3 days.

PER SERVING: 207 calories; 2.3 g fat; 0.4 g saturated fat; 9.8% calories from fat; 0 mg cholesterol; 6.6 g protein; 40.3 g carbohydrate; 1.9 g sugar; 5.8 g fiber; 192 mg sodium; 18 mg calcium; 1.8 mg iron; 16.1 mg vitamin C; 35 mcg beta-carotene; 0.1 mg vitamin E

Rice and Carrot Pilaf

The pineapple in this recipe adds vitamin C and manganese. Pineapple also contains an enzyme called bromelain, which helps to digest food by breaking down protein. This dish tastes equally good hot or cold, so you may want to make extra so you can have it both ways. The rice in this recipe is cooked like pasta, in a generous quantity of water, so you'll need to taste test the rice to determine when it's done. You'll find brown basmati or jasmine rice at natural food stores and well-stocked supermarkets.

4 cups boiling water

1 cup brown basmati or jasmine rice

2 cups carrots, cut into fine matchsticks

1 cup small pineapple chunks, or 1 can (8 ounces) pineapple tidbits, drained

2 tablespoons salted dry-roasted peanuts, coarsely chopped

1 tablespoon freshly squeezed lemon juice

½ teaspoon peeled and grated fresh ginger

1 teaspoon salt

1. Combine the boiling water and rice in a medium saucepan. Lower the heat, cover, and cook for 25 to 35 minutes, until the rice is just tender. Do not overcook. Taste the rice to determine when it's tender. Pour into a strainer to drain the excess water. (If you wish, put a bowl under the strainer and save the water for making soup or cooking beans.)

2. While the rice is cooking, steam the carrots for about 3 minutes, until just barely tender. Transfer to a bowl and add the cooked rice, pineapple, peanuts, lemon juice, and ginger.

3. Season with salt to taste and toss to mix. Serve warm or chilled.

4. Stored in a covered container in the refrigerator, leftover Rice and Carrot Pilaf will keep for up to 2 days.

PER SERVING: 242 calories; 3.8 g fat; 0.6 g saturated fat; 14.2% calories from fat; 0 mg cholesterol; 5.7 g protein; 47.2 g carbohydrate; 8.3 g sugar; 7.7 g fiber; 668 mg sodium; 42 mg calcium; 1.1 mg iron; 6.4 mg vitamin C; 4690 mcg beta-carotene; 1 mg vitamin E

Tex-Mex Bulgur Pilaf

T his colorful bulgur pilaf is influenced by traditions on both sides of the border. The red bell pepper adds wonderful flavor and a healthful dose of beta-carotene and vitamin C. Serve it with Three Bean Chili (page 132) and a crisp salad.

1 cup bulgur

½ teaspoon salt

2 cups boiling water

¼ cup vegetable broth or water

2 tablespoons soy sauce

1 teaspoon chili powder

½ teaspoon ground cumin

½ cup diced red bell pepper

½ cup fresh or frozen green peas

½ cup fresh or frozen corn

1 green onion, thinly sliced

1. Place the bulgur and salt in a saucepan or heatproof bowl. Add the boiling water and stir to mix. Cover and let stand for about 25 minutes, or until the bulgur is tender and the water has been absorbed. The bulgur should be tender but not mushy. Fluff with a fork.

2. Heat the vegetable broth in a nonstick skillet over medium heat. Add the bulgur, soy sauce, chili powder, and cumin. Toss gently with a spatula to mix. Continue cooking, turning with a spatula, until the mixture is very hot and steaming.

3. Gently mix in the bell pepper, peas, corn, and green onion. Reduce the heat to low, cover, and cook for 3 to 5 minutes, until evenly heated through. Serve hot or at room temperature.

4. Stored in a covered container in the refrigerator, leftover Tex-Mex Bulgur Pilaf will keep for up to 3 days.

PER SERVING: 162 calories; 0.9 g fat; 0.1 g saturated fat; 4.7% calories from fat; 0 mg cholesterol; 6.5 g protein; 35.4 g carbohydrate; 3.4 g sugar; 8.1 g fiber; 841 mg sodium; 29 mg calcium; 1.7 mg iron; 34.7 mg vitamin C; 781 mcg beta-carotene; 0.6 mg vitamin E

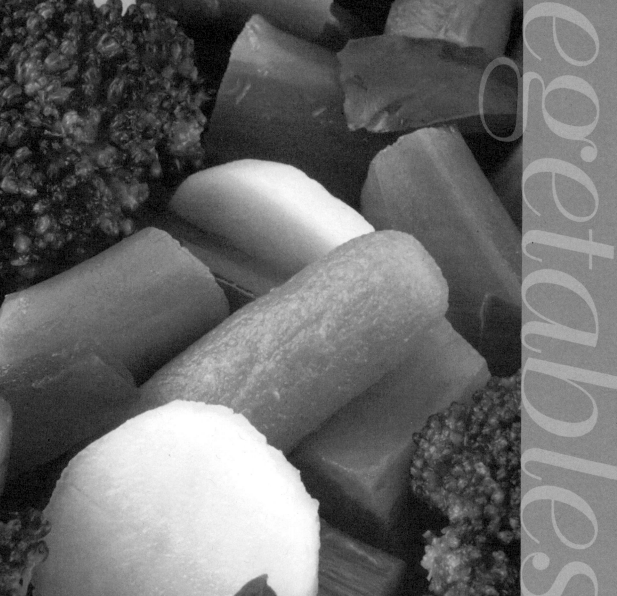

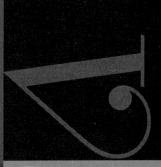

Vegetables

Asian Persuasion Coleslaw

T his salad is a rainbow of gorgeous colors, and its flavorful gingery dressing will keep you coming back for "just one more taste." The cabbage in this recipe adds numerous nutritional benefits and contains a group of cancer-fighting compounds called indoles, which can help fight off breast cancer cells.

2 cups finely shredded green cabbage

2 cups finely shredded red cabbage

1 carrot, shredded or cut into matchsticks

½ cup thinly sliced celery

½ cup finely diced sweet onion

½ cup minced fresh cilantro

2 tablespoons dry-roasted peanuts

2 tablespoons raw sesame seeds

¼ cup seasoned rice vinegar

2 tablespoons apple juice concentrate

1 tablespoon soy sauce

1 tablespoon peeled and minced fresh ginger

1 garlic clove, minced or pressed

¼ teaspoon ground black pepper

1. To make the salad, combine the green cabbage, red cabbage, carrot, celery, onion, cilantro, and peanuts in a large bowl.

2. Toast the sesame seeds in a heavy skillet over high heat for about 2 minutes, stirring constantly, until they begin to pop and become fragrant. Cool, then grind them in a blender or food processor and add to the salad.

3. To make the dressing, combine the vinegar, apple juice concentrate, soy sauce, ginger, garlic, and pepper in a small bowl. Just before serving, pour the dressing over the salad and toss until evenly distributed.

4. This salad is best served immediately. If you must make Asian Persuasion Coleslaw in advance, store the prepared vegetables in a covered container for up to 1 day and toss with the dressing just before serving.

PER SERVING: 87 calories; 3.4 g fat; 0.5 g saturated fat; 35.1% calories from fat; 0 mg cholesterol; 2.6 g protein; 13.6 g carbohydrate; 8.4 g sugar; 2.5 g fiber; 362 mg sodium; 41 mg calcium; 0.9 mg iron; 23.2 mg vitamin C; 841 mcg beta-carotene; 0.4 mg vitamin E

Braised Kale

K ale is a good source of calcium and several phytochemicals that are known to fight cancer. There are many different varieties of kale, each with its own distinctive texture and flavor. A variety of curly green kale is widely available in grocery stores. Two favorites that aren't as common are red Russian and lacinato; these are mainly sold at natural food stores, farmers' markets, and specialty supermarkets. For a slightly different flavor, substitute collard greens for the kale for a traditional Southern favorite.

1 large bunch kale (about 1 pound)

¼ cup water or vegetable broth

3 to 4 garlic cloves, minced or thinly sliced

2 tablespoons soy sauce, or ½ teaspoon salt

1. Wash the kale thoroughly and remove any tough stems. Cut or tear the leaves into small pieces. Set aside.

2. Heat the water in a large skillet. Add the garlic and cook and stir over medium-high heat for about 1 minute, until it begins to soften. Do not let the garlic brown.

3. Lower the heat to medium and stir in the kale. Sprinkle with the soy sauce, if using. Cover and cook for 3 to 5 minutes, stirring frequently. Add extra water, 1 tablespoon at a time, if the kale begins to stick. The kale is done when it is bright green and tender. If you are using salt instead of soy sauce, transfer the kale to a serving dish, sprinkle it with the salt, and toss to mix. Serve at once.

4. Stored in a covered container in the refrigerator, leftover Braised Kale will keep for up to 2 days.

PER SERVING: 40 calories; 0.5 g fat; 0.1 g saturated fat; 10.1% calories from fat; 0 mg cholesterol; 2.8 g protein; 7.9 g carbohydrate; 1.2 g sugar; 2.3 g fiber; 633 mg sodium; 84 mg calcium; 1.2 mg iron; 44.6 mg vitamin C; 8700 mcg beta-carotene; 0.9 mg vitamin E

Broccoli or Cauliflower with Sesame Salt

B roccoli is perfectly cooked when it is brilliant green and tender-crisp. Remove it from the heat at once and serve it right away. Cauliflower is also done cooking when it is tender-crisp. Both are delicious with sesame salt. Unhulled sesame seeds (sometimes called brown sesame seeds) are sold at natural food stores and some supermarkets. Although sesame seeds are high in fat and should be consumed in moderation, they can serve as a great source of calcium and dietary fiber.

1 tablespoon raw unhulled sesame seeds

⅛ teaspoon salt

1 bunch broccoli or cauliflower

1. To make sesame salt, toast the sesame seeds in a heavy skillet over medium heat, stirring constantly, until they begin to pop and brown slightly, about 5 minutes. Transfer to a blender or coffee grinder. Add the salt and grind into a uniform powder.

2. Cut or break the broccoli or cauliflower into bite-size florets. You should have about 4 cups. Peel the broccoli stems and cut them into bite-size pieces. Steam over boiling water or cook in a microwave until just tender. Transfer to a serving bowl and sprinkle with the sesame salt. Toss until evenly distributed. Serve immediately.

3. Stored in a covered container in the refrigerator, leftover Broccoli or Cauliflower with Sesame Salt will keep for up to 2 days.

Variation: Use flaxseeds or black sesame seeds instead of unhulled sesame seeds. If using flaxseeds, do not toast them before grinding.

PER SERVING: 41 calories; 1.2 g fat; 0.2 g saturated fat; 26.3% calories from fat; 0 mg cholesterol; 3.5 g protein; 6 g carbohydrate; 1.7 g sugar; 3.4 g fiber; 85 mg sodium; 56 mg calcium; 1 mg iron; 40.8 mg vitamin C; 674 mcg beta-carotene; 1.4 mg vitamin E

Calabacitas

This recipe is from a burrito shop in Ithaca, New York. The zucchini adds folate and vitamins A and C. Sometimes the shop adds lima beans as well. It's a perfect vegetable combination for tostadas, tacos, or burritos, or it can be used as a side dish or as a baked potato topping.

1 small yellow onion, finely chopped

2 tablespoons water

2 small zucchini, quartered lengthwise and sliced

8 ounces mushrooms, sliced

½ teaspoon ground cumin

½ teaspoon chili powder

1½ cups frozen corn

¼ teaspoon salt

¼ teaspoon ground black pepper

1. Cook the onion in 1 tablespoon of the water, stirring frequently, until the liquid has evaporated. Add the zucchini, mushrooms, and the remaining tablespoon of water. Stir in the cumin and chili powder and simmer for 5 minutes, until the mushrooms are soft.

2. Stir in the corn and cook for 2 minutes longer, until heated through. Season with salt and pepper to taste. Serve immediately.

3. Stored in a covered container in the refrigerator, leftover Calabacitas will keep for up to 3 days.

PER SERVING: 75 calories; 0.7 g fat; 0.1 g saturated fat; 8.8% calories from fat; 0 mg cholesterol; 3 g protein; 17.3 g carbohydrate; 3.6 g sugar; 3.3 g fiber; 154 mg sodium; 18 mg calcium; 1.4 mg iron; 6.9 mg vitamin C; 320 mcg beta-carotene; 0.2 mg vitamin E

Collard Greens with Almonds

ollards are a great source of highly absorbable calcium, and, along with other members of the cruciferous vegetable family (broccoli, brussels sprouts, cauliflower, kale, and rutabaga), they've been shown to be especially helpful in eliminating excess estrogen from a woman's body and reducing breast cancer risk.

¼ cup slivered almonds

1 large bunch collard greens (about 1 pound), rinsed

1 tablespoon rice vinegar

1 small garlic clove, minced or pressed

1. Toast the almonds in a small dry skillet over medium heat for 1 to 2 minutes, until golden. Remove from the skillet and set aside.

2. To remove the stems from the collard greens, work with one leaf at a time. Hold the stem end in one hand and strip the leaf away from the stem with the other hand.

3. Layer 5 collard leaves on a cutting board, roll them into a tight cylinder (like a cigar), and slice them crosswise into thin strips. Repeat until all of the leaves are sliced.

4. Pour 2 inches of water into a large saucepan and bring to a boil over high heat. Add the collard greens, cover, and steam for 4 minutes. Drain and transfer to a bowl.

5. Whisk together the vinegar and garlic in a small bowl until blended. Pour the vinegar mixture over the collard greens just before serving and garnish with the toasted almonds. Serve hot.

PER SERVING: 44 calories; 2.5 g fat; 0.2 g saturated fat; 51.7% calories from fat; 0 mg cholesterol; 2.4 g protein; 4.3 g carbohydrate; 1.2 g sugar; 2.4 g fiber; 11 mg sodium; 103 mg calcium; 1 mg iron; 11.9 mg vitamin C; 3124 mcg beta-carotene; 1.7 mg vitamin E

Garlic Mashed Potatoes

MAKES ABOUT 4 CUPS (4 SERVINGS)

Garlic is a great way to add flavor to mashed potatoes without adding fat. Plus, garlic is rich in selenium, a strong cancer-fighting agent.

5 whole garlic cloves, peeled

2 large russet potatoes, peeled and cut into ½-inch chunks

½ cup water

¼ to ½ cup fortified plain unsweetened soymilk or other nondairy milk

½ teaspoon salt

1. Place the garlic in a medium saucepan. Arrange the potatoes over the garlic. Add the water and bring to a simmer over medium heat. Reduce the heat to low, cover, and cook for about 25 minutes, until the potatoes are tender when pierced with a knife. Check occasionally and add more water, 1 tablespoon at at time, if the saucepan becomes too dry.

2. Mash with a potato masher or fork. Then stir in enough soymilk to obtain a creamy consistency. Season with salt to taste.

3. Stored in a covered container in the refrigerator, leftover Garlic Mashed Potatoes will keep for up to 2 days.

PER SERVING: 143 calories; 0.4 g fat; 0.1 g saturated fat; 2.6% calories from fat; 0 mg cholesterol; 3.3 g protein; 32.3 g carbohydrate; 1.2 g sugar; 3.3 g fiber; 312 mg sodium; 38 mg calcium; 0.7 mg iron; 12.3 mg vitamin C; 3 mcg beta-carotene; 0.2 mg vitamin E

Grilled Plantains

MAKES 4 SERVINGS

While technically a fruit, starchy plantains are often treated like potatoes in cooking. Plantains can be used at any stage of ripeness. They contain folate, a nutrient that plays an important role in cancer prevention.

4 plantains (green, yellow, or speckled)

1. Preheat the oven to 350 degrees F, or heat the grill on medium-high heat. Trim the ends off the plantains and slice each plantain sharply on the diagonal into 2-inch pieces. Bake or grill the plantains for about 10 minutes, until the skins are charred and the flesh is soft. Serve the plantains immediately, in their skins. (The skins aren't edible.)

2. Stored in a covered container in the refrigerator, leftover Grilled Plantains will keep for up to 2 days.

PER SERVING: 278 calories; 0.4 g fat; 0.2 g saturated fat; 1.4% calories from fat; 0 mg cholesterol; 1.9 g protein; 74.8 g carbohydrate; 13.4 g sugar; 5.5 g fiber; 12 mg sodium; 5 mg calcium; 1.4 mg iron; 26.2 mg vitamin C; 886 mcg beta-carotene; 0.3 mg vitamin E

Parsnip Mashed Potatoes

These are the most delicious mashed potatoes, and they're nearly fat free. The garlic in this recipe adds flavor and many health benefits. Garlic contains two main medicinal compounds—allicin and diallyl sulfides—which can help boost the immune system and fight off cancer

3 whole garlic cloves, peeled

1 parsnip, peeled and cut into 1-inch chunks

2 large russet potatoes, peeled and cut into 1-inch chunks

¾ cup water

½ cup fortified plain unsweetened soymilk or other nondairy milk

½ teaspoon salt

⅛ teaspoon ground black pepper

1. Place the garlic in a medium saucepan. Arrange the parsnip over the garlic. Then arrange the potatoes over the parsnip. Add the water and bring to a simmer over medium heat. Reduce the heat to low, cover, and cook for about 25 minutes, until the parsnips and potatoes are tender when pierced with a knife. Check occasionally and add more water, 1 tablespoon at at time, if the saucepan becomes too dry.

2. Mash with a potato masher or fork. Then stir in enough soymilk to obtain a creamy consistency. Season with salt and pepper to taste.

3. Stored in a covered container in the refrigerator, leftover Parsnip Mashed Potatoes will keep for up to 2 days.

PER SERVING: 161 calories; 0.6 g fat; 0.1 g saturated fat; 3.4% calories from fat; 0 mg cholesterol; 4.1 g protein; 36.1 g carbohydrate; 3 g sugar; 4.3 g fiber; 328 mg sodium; 63 mg calcium; 0.9 mg iron; 15.1 mg vitamin C; 3 mcg beta-carotene; 0.3 mg vitamin E

Rutabaga Mashed Potatoes

If you've never cooked with rutabagas, this is a good place to start: a simple recipe with a delicious result. Rutabagas—members of the cruciferous vegetable family along with broccoli, brussels sprouts, cauliflower, radishes, and turnips—are extremely high in vitamin C. They also have generous amounts of many cancer-fighting compounds.

1 medium rutabaga, peeled and cut into ½-inch chunks

2 medium russet potatoes, peeled and cut into ½-inch chunks

1 cup water

½ to 1 cup fortified plain unsweetened soymilk or other nondairy milk

¼ to ½ teaspoon salt

Ground black pepper

1. Arrange the rutabaga in a medium saucepan. Arrange the potatoes over the rutabaga. Add the water and bring to a simmer over medium heat. Reduce the heat to low, cover, and cook for about 25 minutes, until the rutabaga and potatoes are tender when pierced with a knife. Check occasionally and add more water, 1 tablespoon at at time, if the saucpan becomes too dry.

2. Mash with a potato masher or fork. Then stir in enough soymilk to obtain a creamy consistency. Season with salt and pepper to taste.

3. Stored in a covered container in the refrigerator, leftover Rutabaga Mashed Potatoes will keep for up to 2 days.

PER SERVING: 123 calories; 0.8 g fat; 0.1 g saturated fat; 5.7% calories from fat; 0 mg cholesterol; 3.7 g protein; 26.7 g carbohydrate; 3.2 g sugar; 3.7 g fiber; 187 mg sodium; 87 mg calcium; 1 mg iron; 23.2 mg vitamin C; 3 mcg beta-carotene; 0.7 mg vitamin E

Spaghetti Squash with Sauce

Cooked spaghetti squash has a threadlike texture similar to spaghetti, but it is much higher in fiber and anticancer compounds.

1 large spaghetti squash

2 cups fat-free spaghetti sauce

2 tablespoons chopped fresh basil

2 tablespoons nutritional yeast flakes or vegan Parmesan cheese (optional)

Thinly sliced radishes (optional)

1. Preheat the oven to 350 degrees F. Wash the outside of the squash and carefully puncture it with a fork in 5 different places. Place on a baking sheet and bake for 30 to 40 minutes, until tender when pierced with a knife. Set aside to cool. Do not turn off the oven.

2. Cut the cooled squash in half lengthwise and scoop out the seeds with a spoon. Remove the spaghetti-like threads with a fork and place them in a 9-inch round or similar baking dish. Add the spaghetti sauce and toss until it is evenly distributed. Cover lightly with aluminum foil and bake for 20 to 30 minutes, or until heated through.

3. Sprinkle with the basil and optional nutritional yeast. Garnish with radishes, if desired.

4. Stored in a covered container in the refrigerator, leftover Spaghetti Squash with Sauce will keep for up to 2 days.

PER SERVING: 48 calories; 0.3 g fat; 0.1 g saturated fat; 4.6% calories from fat; 0 mg cholesterol; 0.9 g protein; 11.7 g carbohydrate; 8.4 g sugar; 1.6 g fiber; 274 mg sodium; 25 mg calcium; 0.5 mg iron; 6 mg vitamin C; 205 mcg beta-carotene; 0.4 mg vitamin E

Spicy Black Beans and Tomatoes

This is another very low-fat and filling dish. Serve it over brown rice or couscous, scoop it up with baked tortilla chips, or wrap it up in a tortilla.

¼ cup vegetable broth

½ small onion, diced

2 garlic cloves, minced or pressed

½ teaspoon ground cumin

½ teaspoon crushed red pepper flakes

¼ teaspoon chili powder

3 cups cooked or canned black beans, rinsed and drained

2 cans (14.5 ounces each) diced tomatoes, drained, or 3 cups diced fresh tomatoes

2 tablespoons fresh or canned minced green chiles

1 tablespoon minced fresh cilantro or parsley

1. Heat the broth in nonstick skillet over medium-high heat. Add the onion and garlic and cook and stir until tender, about 10 minutes.

2. Add the cumin, crushed red pepper flakes, and chili powder and cook and stir for 2 minutes.

3. Add the black beans, tomatoes, and green chiles. Lower the heat and simmer, stirring occasionally, for about 20 minutes, or until the mixture has thickened slightly.

4. Stir in the cilantro and serve.

5. Stored in a covered container in the refrigerator, leftover Spicy Black Beans and Tomatoes will keep for up to 2 days.

PER SERVING: 254 calories; 1.3 g fat; 0.3 g saturated fat; 4.5% calories from fat; 0 mg cholesterol; 14.7 g protein; 49 g carbohydrate; 10.6 g sugar; 11.6 g fiber; 902 mg sodium; 177 mg calcium; 5.9 mg iron; 23.1 mg vitamin C; 269 mcg beta-carotene; 1.8 mg vitamin E

Sure-Fire Roasted Vegetables

Roasting vegetables with a mix of spices is an easy way to get all the healthful nutrients and fiber you need with very little added fat. Serve them as a side dish, as a main dish over your favorite grain, or wrapped up in a tortilla with salsa.

Mixed Vegetable Combo

1 cup chopped broccoli florets

1 cup diced onion

1 cup diced bell peppers

1 cup diced zucchini or yellow squash

1 cup diced eggplant

1 to 3 garlic cloves, minced or pressed

⅓ cup Italian, Mexican, or Indian Seasoning Mix (see page 183)

1½ cups cooked or canned chickpeas or black beans, rinsed and drained

Root Vegetable Combo

1 cup chopped carrots

1 cup chopped sweet potatoes or new potatoes

1 cup peeled and chopped butternut or other winter squash

1 cup peeled and chopped parsnips or rutabaga

1 cup chopped onion

1 to 3 garlic cloves, minced or pressed

⅓ cup Italian, Mexican, or Indian Seasoning Mix (see page 183)

1½ cups cooked or canned chickpeas or black beans, rinsed and drained

1. Preheat the oven to 400 degrees F. Lightly mist a large, shallow baking pan (such as a jelly roll pan) with vegetable oil spray.
2. Select one of the vegetable combos and place the prepared vegetables in a large bowl. Add your choice of seasoning mix and toss until the vegetables are evenly coated. Transfer to the prepared baking pan and spread out in a single layer.
3. Roast in the oven for 10 minutes. Remove the pan from the oven and mist the top of vegetables lightly with vegetable oil spray. Turn the vegetables over and roast for 5 to 10 minutes longer (root vegetables could take up to 30 minutes longer), or until they are evenly tender.
4. Stir in the beans and serve hot from the oven.
5. Stored in a covered container in the refrigerator, leftover Sure-Fire Roasted Vegetables will keep for up to 2 days.

PER SERVING (Mixed Vegetable Combo with Italian Seasoning Mix): 133 calories; 1.8 g fat; 0.2 g saturated fat; 12.2% calories from fat; 0 mg cholesterol; 6.8 g protein; 24.7 g carbohydrate; 3.8 g sugar; 6 g fiber; 206 mg sodium; 67 mg calcium; 2.7 mg iron; 36.3 mg vitamin C; 458 mcg beta-carotene; 0.8 mg vitamin E

PER SERVING (Root Vegetable Combo with Italian Seasoning Mix): 168 calories; 1.9 g fat; 0.2 g saturated fat; 10% calories from fat; 0 mg cholesterol; 6.9 g protein; 33.1 g carbohydrate; 6.6 g sugar; 7.2 g fiber; 227 mg sodium; 90 mg calcium; 2.8 mg iron; 19 mg vitamin C; 5646 mcg beta-carotene; 1.3 mg vitamin E

Italian Seasoning Mix

¼ cup chopped fresh parsley

2 teaspoons dried basil

2 teaspoons dried rosemary

1 teaspoon dried oregano

¼ teaspoon salt

¼ teaspoon ground black pepper

Combine all of the ingredients in a small bowl.

Mexican Seasoning Mix

¼ cup minced fresh cilantro

2 teaspoons ground cumin

1 teaspoon dried basil

1 teaspoon dried rosemary

¼ teaspoon salt

¼ teaspoon ground black pepper

Combine all of the ingredients in a small bowl.

Indian Seasoning Mix

¼ cup minced fresh cilantro

1 teaspoon curry powder

1 teaspoon garam masala

¼ teaspoon salt

¼ teaspoon ground black pepper

Combine all of the ingredients in a small bowl.

Zippy Yams and Collards

Chili paste, lemon juice, and garlic give this recipe a delightful zip, which is a welcome way to eat nutrient-rich vegetables like yams and collards. The collard greens in this recipe add calcium, folate, and B vitamins.

1 large bunch collard greens (about 1 pound), rinsed

¼ cup water or vegetable broth

1 onion, thinly sliced

2 large garlic cloves, minced

2 small yams or sweet potatoes, peeled (if desired) and cut into bite-size chunks

1 tablespoon vegetarian Worcestershire sauce

½ teaspoon Thai chili paste

¼ teaspoon salt

¼ teaspoon ground black pepper

2 tablespoons freshly squeezed lemon juice

1. To remove the stems from the collard greens, work with one leaf at a time. Hold the stem end in one hand and strip the leaf away from the stem with the other hand.

2. Layer 5 collard leaves on a cutting board, roll them into a tight cylinder (like a cigar), and slice them crosswise into thin strips. Repeat until all the leaves are sliced. Set aside.

3. Heat the water in a deep skillet. Add the onion and garlic and cook and stir until the onion is tender, about 10 minutes. Add the yams, stir, and add enough additional water to cover them. Cover and cook for 5 to 10 minutes, until the yams are soft when pierced with a fork. Remove the lid and simmer uncovered until about half of the water has boiled away.

4. Stir in the collard greens, Worcestershire sauce, and chili paste. Cook and stir until the collard greens are soft. Season with salt and pepper to taste. Sprinkle the lemon over the yams and greens just before serving.

5. Stored in a covered container in the refrigerator, leftover Zippy Yams with Collards will keep for up to 3 days.

PER SERVING: 77 calories; 0.5 g fat; 0.1 g saturated fat; 5.5% calories from fat; 0 mg cholesterol; 3.3 g protein; 16.9 g carbohydrate; 6.3 g sugar; 4.4 g fiber; 83 mg sodium; 164 mg calcium; 1.7 mg iron; 28.6 mg vitamin C; 9064 mcg beta-carotene; 1.2 mg vitamin E

MAIN DISHES

Baked Tofu

aking tofu in a marinade is a simple way to infuse it with flavor. Enjoy it as a finger food or snack, or add it to soups, salads, and other prepared dishes. For best results, start with tofu that is firm or extra-firm, and make certain it is fresh by checking the expiration date on the package.

1 pound firm or extra-firm reduced-fat tofu
(see sidebar)

2 tablespoons soy sauce

2 tablespoons water or unsalted vegetable broth

2 teaspoons brown rice syrup or other liquid sweetener

2 teaspoons balsamic vinegar

2 teaspoons minced garlic

1½ teaspoons peeled and grated fresh ginger

¼ teaspoon ground black pepper

1. Preheat the oven to 400 degrees F. Cut the tofu into 4 equal slices and arrange them in a single, tightly packed layer in a 9-inch square or similar baking dish.

2. Combine the soy sauce, water, syrup, vinegar, garlic, ginger, and pepper in a small bowl. Pour evenly over the tofu and bake uncovered for 30 minutes.

3. Stored in a covered container in the refrigerator, leftover Baked Tofu will keep for up to 3 days.

PER SLICE: 155 calories; 8.4 g fat; 1.2 g saturated fat; 48.9% calories from fat; 0 mg cholesterol; 15.5 g protein; 7.8 g carbohydrate; 2.7 g sugar; 0.6 g fiber; 474 mg sodium; 260 mg calcium; 2.8 mg iron; 1 mg vitamin C; 9 mcg beta-carotene; 0 mg vitamin E

How to Make Tofu Firmer

Some tofu that is labeled "firm" is actually quite soft. To make it firmer, line a baking sheet with a clean dish towel. Cut the tofu into 4 slices and arrange it in a single layer on the towel. Cover the tofu with a second clean towel and top with a cutting board. Place several heavy objects (such canned food, books, or jars of beans) on the cutting board. Let stand for 30 minutes before using the tofu in a recipe. Alternatively, slice the tofu and freeze it prior to using to help maintain its texture. Frozen tofu can be put directly into a recipe, but gently press it first between the palms of your hands to remove excess liquid.

Any Veggie Coconut Curry

T he vegetables listed in this recipes are favorites, but any vegetables you have on hand can be used. Cauliflower, squash, and sweet potatoes are other tasty choices. This is a great way to use up any fresh or frozen vegetables you have on hand. If you decide to use coconut milk, it is important to note that it has a high fat content and should be used in moderation. Use lite coconut milk to get the sweet, nutty coconut flavor without all the fat. Serve this dish over rice or your favorite whole grain.

¼ cup vegetable broth or water

3 large carrots, sliced or diced

1 large onion, diced

4 garlic cloves, minced or pressed

1½ tablespoons curry powder

1 teaspoon ground cumin

½ teaspoon ground turmeric

Pinch of cayenne

3 cups stemmed and chopped kale

2 cups chopped broccoli florets, or 1 package (10 ounces) frozen chopped broccoli

1 medium potato, peeled (if desired) and diced

1½ cups cooked or canned chickpeas, rinsed and drained

1 cup fresh or frozen green peas

8 mushrooms, sliced

1 cup lite coconut milk, or 1 cup plain unsweetened soymilk plus 1 teaspoon coconut extract

3 cups cooked Brown Rice (page 159), kept hot

3 tablespoons reduced-sodium soy sauce

1. Heat the vegetable broth in a large saucepan. Add the carrots, onion, and garlic and cook and stir over medium-high heat for 10 to 15 minutes, or until the onion is translucent. Stir in the curry powder, cumin, turmeric, and cayenne. Cook for 2 to 4 minutes, stirring often.

2. Add the kale, broccoli, potato, chickpeas, green peas, mushrooms, and coconut milk. Cover and lower the heat to medium-low. Simmer for 10 to 20 minutes, stirring occasionally, until the potato can be pierced easily with a fork. Serve over the hot rice. Sprinkle with the soy sauce just before serving.

3. Stored in a covered container in the refrigerator, leftover Any Veggie Coconut Curry will keep for up to 3 days.

PER SERVING: 320 calories; 5.2 g fat; 2.5 g saturated fat; 14.7% calories from fat; 0 mg cholesterol; 12.3 g protein; 59.3 g carbohydrate; 5.9 g sugar; 12.3 g fiber; 407 mg sodium; 115 mg calcium; 4.7 mg iron; 37.7 mg vitamin C; 6312 mcg beta-carotene; 1.7 mg vitamin E

Broccoli à la King

In this recipe, broccoli and mushrooms are served in a creamy sauce with toasted almonds over rice or pasta. Broccoli is loaded with sulforaphane, which has powerful anticancer activity.

⅓ cup millet

2¼ cups water

¼ cup raw cashews

¼ cup blanched almonds

⅓ cup vegetable broth or water

1 tablespoon soy sauce

1 onion, diced

4 cups sliced mushrooms (about 1 pound)

2 tablespoons dry sherry or vegetable broth

½ teaspoon dried thyme

¼ teaspoon whole celery seeds

¼ teaspoon ground black pepper

3 cups chopped broccoli florets

½ to 1 teaspoon salt

4 cups cooked whole wheat pasta or Brown Rice (page 159), kept hot

1. Combine the millet with 1¼ cups of the water in a saucepan and bring to a boil. Lower the heat, cover, and cook, stirring occasionally, for about 55 minutes, or until the millet is tender and all of the water has been absorbed.

2. Transfer the cooked millet to a blender. Add the cashews and the remaining cup of water. Process for 1 to 2 minutes, until completely smooth. Set aside.

3. Preheat the oven to 350 degrees F.

4. Arrange the almonds in a single layer on a baking sheet and toast them in the oven for about 12 minutes, until lightly browned and fragrant. Cool. Coarsely chop the almonds by hand or in a food processor. Set aside.

5. Combine the vegetable broth and soy sauce in a large skillet. Add the onion and cook and stir over medium-high heat for about 5 minutes, until the onion is soft. Reduce the heat to medium and add the mushrooms, sherry, thyme, celery seeds, and pepper. Stir to mix. Cover and cook for about 5 minutes, stirring occasionally, until the mushrooms are tender. If needed, add 1 to 2 tablespoons of additional sherry or vegetable broth to prevent sticking.

6. Stir in the millet mixture, broccoli, and almonds. Cover and cook over medium-low heat for about 5 minutes, stirring occasionally, until the broccoli is just tender. Season with salt to taste. Serve over the hot pasta.

7. Stored in a covered container in the refrigerator, leftover Broccoli à la King will keep for up to 3 days.

PER SERVING: 196 calories; 5.1 g fat; 0.7 g saturated fat; 23.5% calories from fat; 0 mg cholesterol; 8.1 g protein; 31.7 g carbohydrate; 2.2 g sugar; 5.1 g fiber; 306 mg sodium; 42 mg calcium; 2.3 mg iron; 14.6 mg vitamin C; 219 mcg beta-carotene; 1.8 mg vitamin E

Buckwheat Pasta with Seitan

This recipe contains soba noodles, a Japanese buckwheat pasta. Buckwheat is a great source of rutin, a type of bioflavonoid that has an amazing capacity to fight free radicals, which are responsible for many cancers. Soba noodles are available at Asian markets and may also be found in the Asian food section of many supermarkets and natural food stores. Whole wheat angel hair pasta or spaghetti can be used as an alternative to the soba noodles, if you prefer.

12 ounces soba noodles

1¾ cups vegetable broth or water

1 medium onion, thinly sliced

3 cups sliced fresh mushrooms

1 red bell pepper, sliced

1 yellow bell pepper, sliced

8 ounces seitan, sliced

2 tablespoons flour (any kind)

2 teaspoons soy sauce

1 teaspoon chopped garlic, or ½ teaspoon garlic powder

¼ teaspoon ground black pepper

Salt

¼ cup chopped fresh parsley

1. Cook the soba noodles in a large pot of boiling water until just tender, about 8 minutes or according to the package directions. Drain and rinse with cold water to prevent them from sticking. Set aside.

2. Heat ¼ cup of the vegetable broth in a large skillet. Add the onion and cook and stir until the onion is transparent, about 10 minutes. Add the mushrooms and bell peppers. Cover and cook for 5 to 10 minutes, until the mushrooms and peppers are tender. Stir in the seitan. Add a small amount of water if the pan becomes dry.

3. Whisk together the flour and the remaining 1½ cups of vegetable broth until smooth. Stir into the seitan mixture along with the soy sauce, garlic, pepper, and salt to taste. Cook and stir over medium-low heat until thickened.

4. Pour the seitan mixture over the soba noodles. Garnish with the parsley and serve.

5. Stored in a covered container in the refrigerator, leftover Buckwheat Pasta with Seitan will keep for 2 to 3 days.

Note: Most brands of soba noodles contain sodium. Try to find a brand that is lower in sodium and consider omitting salt from the cooking water.

PER SERVING: 263 calories; 1.3 g fat; 0.2 g saturated fat; 4.4% calories from fat; 0 mg cholesterol; 17.6 g protein; 49.5 g carbohydrate; 4.9 g sugar; 5.6 g fiber; 796 mg sodium; 53 mg calcium; 3.1 mg iron; 67 mg vitamin C; 751 mcg beta-carotene; 0.9 mg vitamin E

Easy Stir-Fry

D inner was never so easy! While not considered gourmet, frozen vegetables are often as nutrient rich as fresh vegetables, and sometimes even more so, because they are frozen at their peak of freshness.

1 bag (16 ounces) **frozen stir-fry vegetables**

1½ cups cooked or canned beans (your favorite kind), **rinsed and drained**

¼ cup low-fat stir-fry sauce

2 cups cooked Couscous (page 163), **Brown Rice** (page 159), **or other whole grain, kept hot**

1. Cook and stir the vegetables in a nonstick pan over medium-high heat with 2 to 3 tablespoons of water as needed. Once the vegetables have thawed but are not completely cooked, add the beans and sauce. Cook and stir over medium heat until the vegetables are tender-crisp.

2. Serve over the hot couscous or cooked grain of your choice.

3. Stored in a covered container in the refrigerator, leftover Easy Stir-Fry will keep for up to 3 days.

PER SERVING: 299 calories; 1.5 g fat; 0.3 g saturated fat; 4.6% calories from fat; 0 mg cholesterol; 14.4 g protein; 57.1 g carbohydrate; 4.9 g sugar; 10.9 g fiber; 1067 mg sodium; 103 mg calcium; 4.2 mg iron; 3.5 mg vitamin C; 2291 mcg beta-carotene; 1.3 mg vitamin E

Eggplant Lasagne

ender slices of eggplant take the place of pasta in this lasagne, making it quite high in fiber. This recipe includes many flavorful and healthful spices and herbs, including oregano, a powerful source of antioxidants. This dish can be assembled ahead of time and baked just before serving. Serve it with polenta or sourdough bread and a green salad.

1 large eggplant, unpeeled

3½ cups bottled marinara sauce or Simple Marinara (page 156)

1½ cups water

1 large onion, diced

4 pounds chopped fresh spinach, or 2 packages (10 ounces each) frozen chopped spinach, thawed

2 teaspoons dried basil

1 teaspoon dried oregano

½ teaspoon salt

½ teaspoon garlic powder

¼ teaspoon ground nutmeg

¼ cup whole wheat flour

1 teaspoon soy sauce (optional)

3 garlic cloves, minced or pressed

4 cups sliced mushrooms

1 teaspoon dried thyme

¼ teaspoon ground black pepper

1. Preheat the oven to 375 degrees F. Lightly mist a baking sheet with vegetable oil spray.

2. Cut the eggplant into ¼-inch-thick slices (there should be about 12 slices) and arrange them in a single layer on the prepared baking sheet. Bake for 20 minutes, turn the slices over, and bake for 15 minutes longer. The eggplant should be tender when pierced with a fork. Remove from the oven and lower the oven temperature to 350 degrees F.

3. Spread half of the marinara sauce in a 9-inch square casserole or baking dish and arrange half of the eggplant slices over it.

4. Heat ½ cup of the water in a large nonstick skillet. Add the onion and cook and stir over high heat until all of the liquid has evaporated. Add another ¼ cup of the water and stir to loosen any stuck bits of onion. Continue to cook and stir until all of the liquid evaporates again. Repeat this process 2 more times.

5. Lower the heat to medium and add the spinach, basil, oregano, salt, garlic powder, and nutmeg. Cook for about 3 minutes, stirring often, until the spinach is hot. Stir in the flour and cook for 2 minutes longer, stirring constantly. Spread half of the spinach mixture evenly over the eggplant slices.

6. Heat the remaining ¼ cup of water and the optional soy sauce in a large nonstick skillet. Add the garlic and cook and stir for 1 minute. Add the mushrooms, thyme, and pepper. Cook for about 5 minutes over medium heat, stirring often, until the mushrooms are tender. Carefully spread the mushroom mixture over the spinach.

7. Arrange the remaining eggplant slices over the mushroom mixture and spread the remaining spinach over the eggplant. Pour the remaining marinara sauce on top.

8. Bake uncovered for about 40 minutes, or until heated through.

9. Stored in a covered container in the refrigerator, leftover Eggplant Lasagne will keep for up to 3 days.

PER SERVING: 107 calories; 1 g fat; 0.2 g saturated fat; 8% calories from fat; 0 mg cholesterol; 5.4 g protein; 23.6 g carbohydrate; 8.5 g sugar; 6.8 g fiber; 715 mg sodium; 110 mg calcium; 3.1 mg iron; 11.8 mg vitamin C; 3645 mcg beta-carotene; 4.2 mg vitamin E

Home-Style Squash and Pinto Beans

Vegetables, rice, and beans make this all-American dish a welcome repast after a hard day. This recipe contains 12 grams of fiber and less than 2 grams of fat. Serve it with a salad and fruit wedges.

¼ to ½ cup vegetable broth, as needed

½ cup diced onion

2 teaspoons seeded and minced jalapeño chile

2 garlic cloves, minced or pressed

1 cup sliced yellow squash (½-inch-thick slices)

1 cup sliced zucchini (½-inch-thick slices)

1½ cups cooked or canned pinto beans, rinsed and drained

1 can (14.5 ounces) diced tomatoes, undrained, or 1½ cups chopped fresh tomatoes plus ½ cup tomato juice, water, or vegetable broth

½ cup fresh or frozen corn kernels

3 fresh thyme sprigs

2 cups cooked Brown Rice (page 159), Couscous (page 163), or pasta, kept hot

1. Heat ¼ cup of the vegetable broth in a large skillet over medium-high heat. Add the onion, chile, and garlic and cook and stir for 2 minutes.

2. Stir in the squash and zucchini and cook and stir for 2 minutes. Add the beans, tomatoes and their liquid, corn, and thyme sprigs. Lower the heat, cover, and simmer for 10 minutes.

3. Remove and discard the thyme sprigs. Serve over the hot rice.

4. Stored in a covered container in the refrigerator, leftover Home-Style Squash and Pinto Beans will keep for up to 3 days.

PER SERVING: 268 calories; 1.9 g fat; 0.3 g saturated fat; 6.4% calories from fat; 0 mg cholesterol; 11.6 g protein; 53.6 g total carbohydrate; 5.6 g sugar; 11.9 g fiber; 323 mg sodium; 91 mg calcium; 3.4 mg iron; 14.9 mg vitamin C; 270 mcg beta-carotene; 1.6 mg vitamin E

Lazy Lasagne

Your days of preparing complicated, high-fat lasagne are over. This version uses uncooked lasagne noodles, which makes it extra-easy to prepare. Enjoy this cholesterol- and dairy-free meal, which also boasts plenty of filling fiber and cancer-fighting nutrients. Top this dish with a generous sprinkling of fortified nutritional yeast for a cheesier flavor and added vitamin B_{12}.

3 pounds fresh spinach, cleaned and chopped, or 1 bag (16 ounces) **frozen chopped spinach, thawed**

1 pound firm reduced-fat tofu, mashed

4 garlic cloves, minced or pressed

1 teaspoon salt

2 cans (28 ounces each) tomato sauce

1 pound whole wheat lasagna noodles

10 button mushrooms, sliced, or 3 cups chopped vegetables (your favorites)

10 fresh basil leaves, thinly sliced, or 1 teaspoon dried basil

1 teaspoon dried oregano

¼ cup vegan Parmesan cheese or nutritional yeast flakes

1. Preheat the oven to 325 degrees F. Combine the spinach, tofu, garlic, and salt in a large bowl.

2. Pour ½ cup of the tomato sauce over the bottom of a 9 x 13-inch baking pan. Arrange a layer of the lasagna noodles over the sauce, overlapping the noodles slightly. Spread half of the spinach and tofu mixture on top of the lasagna noodles, and cover the spinach and tofu layer with another layer of lasagna noodles. Add a layer of some of the tomato sauce, enough to cover the noodles, and then add a layer of the mushrooms. Sprinkle half of the basil and ½ teaspoon of the oregano evenly over the mushrooms. Continue to add layers of noodles, spinach and tofu, noodles, tomato sauce, mushrooms, and the remaining basil and oregano until the layers reach the top of the pan. The final layer should be sauce. Sprinkle the vegan Parmesan cheese evenly over the top.

3. Cover tightly with aluminum foil and bake for 1 hour. Uncover and stick a knife through the center of the lasagne to make sure the noodles are completely cooked. Uncover and let cool for 15 minutes before serving.

4. Stored in a covered container in the refrigerator, leftover Lazy Lasagne will keep for up to 3 days.

PER SERVING: 334 calories; 4.6 g fat; 0.7 g saturated fat; 12.4% calories from fat; 0 mg cholesterol; 18.4 g protein; 62.8 g carbohydrate; 10.3 g sugar; 11 g fiber; 1449 mg sodium; 147 mg calcium; 6.3 mg iron; 16.9 mg vitamin C; 3152 mcg beta-carotene; 6.2 mg vitamin E

Mushroom Stroganoff over Fettuccine

This hearty stroganoff is made with seitan, a fat-free, high-protein meat alternative made from wheat. Seitan is sometimes called "wheat meat" because of its amazing ability to mimic meat in taste and texture. It is sold in the refrigerated section of natural food stores and many large grocery stores.

1½ cups plus 2 tablespoons water

1 small onion, diced

1 pound cremini or button mushrooms, sliced

6 to 8 garlic cloves, minced

8 ounces seitan, cut into strips

1 cup roasted red bell peppers, chopped

3 tablespoons unsalted tomato paste

2 teaspoons paprika

½ teaspoon ground black pepper

¼ cup raw cashews

1½ cups cooked or canned white beans, rinsed and drained

½ cup bean cooking liquid, water, or vegetable broth

2 tablespoons red wine vinegar or balsamic vinegar

2 teaspoons soy sauce

12 ounces fettuccine

1. Heat ½ cup of the water in a large nonstick skillet. Add the onion and cook and stir over high heat for about 5 minutes, until translucent.

2. Reduce the heat to medium. Stir in the mushrooms, garlic, and 2 more tablespoons of the water. Cover and cook for 5 minutes, stirring occasionally.

3. Add the seitan, bell peppers, tomato paste, paprika, and pepper. Cover and cook over medium-low heat for 5 minutes.

4. Combine the cashews and the remaining cup of water in a blender. Process on high speed until completely smooth, about 2 minutes. Add the beans and the bean cooking liquid and process on high for about 1 minute, until completely smooth. Pour into the skillet with the mushrooms. Add the vinegar and soy sauce and stir until evenly mixed. Heat gently, adding additional water as needed, 1 tablespoon at a time, to achieve the desired consistency.

5. Cook the fettuccine in boiling water until just tender. Drain and rinse under cold water. Top with the mushroom mixture and serve immediately.

6. Stored in a covered container in the refrigerator, leftover Mushroom Stroganoff over Fettuccine will keep for up to 2 days.

PER SERVING: 403 calories; 4.5 g fat; 0.8 g saturated fat; 10% calories from fat; 0 mg cholesterol; 23.4 g protein; 68.9 g carbohydrate; 4.5 g sugar; 8.9 g fiber; 322 mg sodium; 90 mg calcium; 6.5 mg iron; 44.3 mg vitamin C; 789 mcg beta-carotene; 1.6 mg vitamin E

No-Meat Loaf

S erve this great-tasting loaf with Garlic Mashed Potatoes (page 177) and Mushroom Gravy (page 156) for a hearty meal that's sure to please. A food processor makes it easy to make fresh bread crumbs (or you can purchase packaged bread crumbs) and to finely chop the walnuts and vegetables. The tomato sauce in this recipe adds vitamin C and lycopene.

1 package (14 ounces) **vegan burger crumbles, or 2 cups cooked Bulgur** (page 162)

1½ cups bread crumbs, preferably whole wheat (2 to 3 slices of bread)

1¼ cups rolled oats (old-fashioned or quick-cooking)

1 cup tomato sauce or crushed tomatoes

1 small onion, minced

2 celery stalks, minced

1 carrot, minced

½ green bell pepper, minced

¼ cup finely chopped walnuts

3 tablespoons reduced-sodium soy sauce

2 teaspoons stone-ground or Dijon mustard

½ teaspoon dried thyme

½ teaspoon dried sage

¼ teaspoon ground black pepper

½ cup ketchup or barbecue sauce (optional)

1. Preheat the oven to 350 degrees F. Lightly mist a 5 x 9-inch loaf pan or similar baking dish with vegetable oil spray.

2. Combine the vegan burger crumbles, bread crumbs, oats, tomato sauce, onion, celery, carrot, bell pepper, walnuts, soy sauce, mustard, thyme, sage, and pepper in a large bowl. Mix with a large spoon or your hands until the mixture is evenly combined.

3. Press into the prepared loaf pan. Spread the optional ketchup over the top and bake for 60 minutes. Let stand for 10 minutes before slicing.

4. To store leftovers, remove the loaf from the pan and let cool. Stored in a covered container in the refrigerator, leftover No-Meat Loaf will keep for up to 3 days.

PER SERVING: 104 calories; 2.6 g fat; 0.3 g saturated fat; 22% calories from fat; 0 mg cholesterol; 8.2 g protein; 13.9 g carbohydrate; 2.7 g sugar; 2.5 g fiber; 418 mg sodium; 37 mg calcium; 1.7 mg iron; 5.9 mg vitamin C; 463 mcg beta-carotene; 0.6 mg vitamin E; 3094 mcg lycopene

Penne with Kale, Tomatoes, and Olives

The kale in this flavorful combination provides highly absorbable calcium and isothiocyanates, which have strong anticancer effects.

¼ cup vegetable broth or water

1 onion, diced

5 cups chopped kale

2 cans (14.5 ounces each) chopped fire-roasted tomatoes, undrained, or 3 cups chopped fresh tomatoes plus ½ cup water or vegetable broth

½ cup sliced kalamata olives

1 tablespoon chopped fresh parsley

8 ounces whole wheat penne

¼ cup vegan Parmesan cheese or nutritional yeast flakes (optional)

1. Heat the vegetable broth in a large saucepan. Add the onion and cook and stir over medium heat for 3 minutes. Add the kale and the tomatoes and their liquid. Bring to a boil, lower the heat, cover, and simmer for 20 minutes. Stir in the olives and parsley and cook for 5 minutes longer.

2. While the kale is cooking, bring a large pot of water to a boil and cook the penne until just tender. Drain and transfer to a serving bowl. Add the kale mixture and toss gently. Sprinkle the top with the optional vegan Parmesan cheese and serve immediately.

3. Stored in a covered container in the refrigerator, leftover Penne with Kale, Tomatoes, and Olives will keep for up to 3 days.

PER SERVING: 281 calories; 3.3 g fat; 0.5 g saturated fat; 10.5% calories from fat; 0 mg cholesterol; 12 g protein; 57.6 g carbohydrate; 8.3 g sugar; 8.7 g fiber; 497 mg sodium; 166 mg calcium; 5 mg iron; 53.9 mg vitamin C; 6796 mcg beta-carotene; 2.9 mg vitamin E

Potato and Cauliflower Curry (Aloo Gobi)

MAKES 6 SERVINGS

Turmeric and other Indian spices are getting more and more attention for their anticancer properties. Combine them with known cancer-fighting vegetables and you're in for real health food. For a hotter curry, increase the amount of cayenne.

1 cup water, as needed

1 onion, diced or thinly sliced

3 to 4 cups cauliflower florets

2 medium potatoes, peeled (if desired) **and diced**

½ teaspoon whole cumin seeds

½ teaspoon ground turmeric

½ teaspoon ground coriander

¼ teaspoon ground ginger

¼ teaspoon ground cinnamon

⅛ to ¼ teaspoon cayenne

1 can (15 ounces) **diced tomatoes, undrained, or** 1½ cups chopped fresh tomatoes

2 tablespoons apple juice concentrate

½ teaspoon salt

1. Heat ½ cup of the water in a large pot. Add the onion and cook and stir over medium-high heat for about 3 minutes, until the onion begins to soften. Lower the heat to medium and add the cauliflower and potatoes. Continue cooking, stirring often, for about 5 minutes. Add more of the water, ¼ cup at a time, as needed to prevent sticking.

2. Toast the cumin seeds, turmeric, coriander, ginger, cinnamon, and cayenne in a dry skillet over medium heat for about 2 minutes, stirring constantly. Add the spices to cauliflower mixture along with the tomatoes and their juice, apple juice concentrate, and salt and stir to mix. Cover and simmer for about 20 minutes, or until the vegetables are tender.

3. Stored in a covered container in the refrigerator, leftover Potato and Cauliflower Curry will keep for up to 3 days.

Variation: For a sweeter curry, add ½ cup of golden raisins along with the tomatoes.

PER SERVING: 91 calories; 0.4 g fat; 0.1 g saturated fat; 4.1% calories from fat; 0 mg cholesterol; 2.7 g protein; 20.9 g carbohydrate; 5.6 g sugar; 3.9 g fiber; 302 mg sodium; 53 mg calcium; 2.3 mg iron; 30 mg vitamin C; 66 mcg beta-carotene; 0.6 mg vitamin E

Quinoa Pilaf

Quinoa can add variety to your diet and contains more protein than other grains.

¼ to ½ cup water

1 yellow or red onion, chopped

½ cup chopped celery

½ cup chopped carrot

1 tablespoon minced garlic

2 cups quinoa, rinsed and drained

2 teaspoons ground cumin

1 teaspoon dried oregano

3 cups boiling water or vegetable broth

1 teaspoon salt (add only if using boiling water or unsalted broth)

¼ cup minced fresh cilantro or parsley (optional)

1. Heat ¼ cup of the water in a large pot. Add the onion, celery, carrot, and garlic and cook and stir until the onion is soft and translucent, about 10 minutes.

2. Add the quinoa, cumin, and oregano and cook and stir for 3 minutes. Add the boiling water and salt, if using, lower the heat, cover, and cook for about 20 minutes, or until all of the liquid has been absorbed and the quinoa has "bloomed." Do not stir the quinoa during cooking, and make sure the lid is tight to prevent moisture from escaping.

3. Remove from the heat and allow the quinoa to rest for 5 to 10 minutes. Add the optional cilantro, fluff with a fork, and serve.

4. Stored in a covered container in the refrigerator, leftover Quinoa Pilaf will keep for up to 3 days.

Variation: Omit the cumin and oregano and add 1 teaspoon dried thyme, rosemary, and/or sage.

PER SERVING: 172 calories; 2.6 g fat; 0.3 g saturated fat; 13.8% calories from fat; 0 mg cholesterol; 6 g protein; 32 g carbohydrate; 3.6 g sugar; 3.1 g fiber; 318 mg sodium; 45 mg calcium; 4.4 mg iron; 1.7 mg vitamin C; 647 mcg beta-carotene; 0.8 mg vitamin E

Red Bean Casserole

This simple casserole is high in fiber, which helps your body eliminate excess hormones, toxins, and carcinogens. Just one serving of this casserole has 8 grams of fiber, so you'll be well on your way to your daily goal of 40 grams.

3 cups cooked long-grain Brown Rice (page 159)

3 cups cooked or canned red beans, rinsed and drained

1 cup diced red onion

1 cup diced celery

2 tablespoons minced fresh parsley

1 teaspoon salt

1 garlic clove, minced or pressed

½ teaspoon ground black pepper

Dash of hot sauce

1. Preheat the oven to 350 degrees F. Lightly mist a 9 x 13-inch baking dish with vegetable oil spray.

2. Combine all of the ingredients in the prepared casserole dish and mix until evenly combined. Bake uncovered for 20 minutes, or until heated through.

3. Stored in a covered container in the refrigerator, leftover Red Bean Casserole will keep for up to 3 days.

PER SERVING: 344 calories; 1.2 g fat; 0.3 g saturated fat; 3.2% calories from fat; 0 mg cholesterol; 15.2 g protein; 68.5 g total carbohydrate; 2.9 g sugar; 8 g fiber; 967 mg sodium; 71 mg calcium; 5.5 mg iron; 6.9 mg vitamin C; 204 mcg beta-carotene; 0.6 mg vitamin E

Sweet-and-Sour Stir-Fry

The celery in this recipe contains the compound luteolin, which has been shown to kill colon cancer cells. If you've ever prepared a stir-fry, you know that once the cooking begins, everything happens very quickly. The secret to a serene stir-fry experience is to prepare the vegetables and mix the sauce ingredients in advance; then arrange everything within easy reach of the stove. Serve this dish with Brown Rice (page 159) or Chinese Fried Bulgur (page 167).

2 tablespoons raw sesame seeds

½ cup crushed pineapple packed in juice

½ cup apple juice concentrate

¼ cup crushed tomatoes or tomato sauce

2 tablespoons soy sauce

2 tablespoons seasoned rice vinegar

1½ teaspoons cornstarch

¼ teaspoon ground black pepper

¼ cup vegetable broth or water

1 onion, thinly sliced

1 cup diagonally sliced celery

1 carrot, diagonally sliced

1 green bell pepper, sliced into strips

¾ cup water

4 or 5 garlic cloves, minced or pressed

2 tablespoons thinly sliced fresh basil, or ½ teaspoon dried basil

2 cups sliced mushrooms

8 ounces seitan, cut into strips

1. Place the sesame seeds in a heavy skillet. Cook and stir over medium heat for 2 to 3 minutes, until the seeds become fragrant and begin to pop. Remove from the skillet and set aside.

2. Combine the pineapple and its juice, apple juice concentrate, tomatoes, soy sauce, vinegar, cornstarch, and pepper in a small bowl. Mix well and set aside.

3. Heat the broth in a wok or large skillet. Add the onion and cook and stir over high heat for 2 to 3 minutes, until just soft.

4. Add the celery, carrot, bell pepper, water, garlic, and basil and cook and stir until the vegetables are tender-crisp, about 2 to 3 minutes. Add the mushrooms and seitan and continue to cook and stir for about 3 minutes longer, until the mushrooms are tender.

5. Stir in the reserved pineapple mixture and continue cooking for about 2 minutes, until the sauce thickens. Transfer to a serving dish and sprinkle with the toasted sesame seeds.

6. Stored in a covered container in the refrigerator, leftover Sweet-and-Sour Stir-Fry will keep for up to 3 days.

PER SERVING: 113 calories; 1.7 g fat; 0.2 g saturated fat; 13.4% calories from fat; 0 mg cholesterol; 7.8 g protein; 18.2 g carbohydrate; 11.5 g sugar; 1.8 g fiber; 353 mg sodium; 40 mg calcium; 1.4 mg iron; 15.9 mg vitamin C; 703 mcg beta-carotene; 0.3 mg vitamin E

Tempeh Broccoli Sauté

Tempeh, which is made from fermented soybeans, is easy to digest and is incredibly high in protein. Just one serving of this recipe contains 20 grams of protein. Plus, the broccoli in this recipe adds highly absorbable calcium, and the whole dish takes just minutes to prepare. For variety, this sauté can be served over Brown Rice (page 159) or your favorite whole grain instead of couscous.

1 package (10 ounces) **tempeh**

¼ cup vegetable broth

2 bunches broccoli, chopped, or 2 bags (16 ounces each) **frozen broccoli florets**

1 small onion, diced

1 red bell pepper, diced

1 tablespoon minced or pressed garlic

1 tablespoon peeled and minced fresh ginger, or 1 teaspoon ground ginger

1 tablespoon soy sauce

2 cups cooked Couscous (page 163), **kept hot**

1. Cut the tempeh into ½-inch cubes and steam for 10 minutes.
2. Heat the broth in a wok or large skillet and add the tempeh, broccoli, onion, bell pepper, garlic, and ginger. Cook and stir over medium-high heat until the tempeh is lightly browned and the vegetables are tender-crisp.
3. Add the soy sauce just before serving. Serve over the hot couscous.
4. Stored in a covered container in the refrigerator, leftover Tempeh Broccoli Sauté will keep for up to 3 days.

PER SERVING: 285 calories; 8.1 g fat; 1.7 g saturated fat; 25.5% calories from fat; 0 mg cholesterol; 20.2 g protein; 37.2 g carbohydrate; 5.8 g sugar; 7.1 g fiber; 312 mg sodium; 127 mg calcium; 3.1 mg iron; 86.4 mg vitamin C; 1293 mcg beta-carotene; 2.3 mg vitamin E

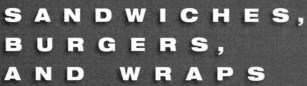

**SANDWICHES,
BURGERS,
AND WRAPS**

Eggless Salad Sandwich

The filling in these sandwiches has the flavor and appearance of egg salad, without the saturated fat and cholesterol.

1 pound firm reduced-fat silken tofu

1 green onion, finely chopped

2 tablespoons pickle relish

2 tablespoons fat-free or low-fat vegan mayonnaise

2 teaspoons yellow mustard

1 teaspoon salt

¼ teaspoon ground cumin

¼ teaspoon ground turmeric

¼ teaspoon garlic powder

12 slices whole-grain bread

6 lettuce leaves

6 tomato slices

1. Mash the tofu with a fork or potato masher, leaving some chunks.

2. Stir in the green onion, relish, mayonnaise, mustard, salt, cumin, turmeric, and garlic powder. Spread on the bread and garnish with the lettuce and tomato.

3. Stored in a covered container in the refrigerator, leftover Eggless Salad (without the bread, lettuce, or tomato) will keep for up to 3 days.

PER SERVING: 175 calories; 3 g fat; 0.6 g saturated fat; 15.6% calories from fat; 0 mg cholesterol; 9.1 g protein; 30.5 g carbohydrate; 8.9 g sugar; 4.4 g fiber; 827 mg sodium; 67 mg calcium; 2.6 mg iron; 3.5 mg vitamin C; 127 mcg beta-carotene; 0.4 mg vitamin E

Chickpea Burgers

T hese tasty golden patties are made with chickpeas, also known as garbanzo beans. Chickpeas have a delicious nutlike taste and texture and are a great source of protein. You can prepare the mixture in no time at all if you use canned beans and chop the ingredients in a food processor. Serve these burgers on whole-grain buns with all the fixings, or try them with Tex-Mex Bulgur Pilaf (page 170) and salsa.

2 tablespoons raw sesame seeds

1 small onion, finely chopped

1 small carrot, finely chopped

1 celery stalk, finely chopped

1 garlic clove, minced or pressed

1½ cups cooked or canned chickpeas, rinsed and drained

½ cup cooked Bulgur (page 162) or Brown Rice (page 159)

1 tablespoon soy sauce

1½ teaspoons curry powder

1 teaspoon ground cumin

½ teaspoon salt

½ teaspoon ground coriander or cardamom

⅛ teaspoon cayenne

¼ cup potato flour, as needed

1. Place the sesame seeds in a heavy skillet. Cook and stir over medium heat for 2 to 3 minutes, until the seeds become fragrant and begin to pop. Grind them in a food processor or blender and transfer to a mixing bowl. Add the onion, carrot, celery, and garlic.

2. Place the beans in a food processor and pulse until chopped. Alternatively, coarsely mash the beans with a potato masher, leaving some chunks. Add the chopped beans to the vegetable mixture along with the cooked bulgur, soy sauce, curry powder, cumin, salt, coriander, and cayenne. Mix thoroughly.

3. Stir in just enough of the potato flour to form a stiff dough. Knead for 30 seconds and form into 6 patties.

4. Lightly mist a nonstick skillet with vegetable oil spray. Cook the patties in the skillet over medium heat for about 2 minutes, until the bottoms are lightly browned. Turn the patties over and cook for 2 minutes longer, until lightly browned. Serve hot.

5. Stored in a covered container in the refrigerator, leftover Chickpea Burgers will keep for up to 3 days.

PER SERVING: 130 calories; 3.2 g fat; 0.4 g saturated fat; 22.5% calories from fat; 0 mg cholesterol; 6 g protein; 20.7 g carbohydrate; 1.3 g sugar; 4.9 g fiber; 430 mg sodium; 45 mg calcium; 2.3 mg iron; 2.2 mg vitamin C; 683 mcg beta-carotene; 0.4 mg vitamin E

Chickpea Salad Romaine Wraps

In this recipe, salad becomes finger food, as leaves of romaine lettuce are used to wrap a tasty chickpea filling. This makes a refreshing wrap that's high in healthful fiber.

1½ cups cooked or canned chickpeas, rinsed and drained

½ cup finely chopped or grated carrot

½ cup finely chopped celery

3 green onions, chopped

2 to 3 tablespoons fat-free or low-fat vegan mayonnaise

1 tablespoon stone-ground mustard

½ teaspoon salt

¼ teaspoon ground black pepper

4 large romaine lettuce leaves

1 medium tomato, sliced, or 6 to 8 cherry tomatoes, cut in half

1. Coarsely mash the beans with a fork or potato masher, leaving some chunks. Add the carrot, celery, green onions, mayonnaise, mustard, salt, and pepper. Mix well.

2. Place about one-quarter of the mixture on each lettuce leaf. Add one-quarter of the tomato, roll the lettuce around the filling, and serve.

3. Stored in a covered container in the refrigerator, leftover Chickpea Salad Romaine Wrap filling (without the lettuce and tomato) will keep for up to 3 days.

Variations

CHICKPEA SALAD SANDWICH: Spread one-third of the chickpea mixture on whole-grain bread. Top with the tomato slices, lettuce leaves, and another slice of bread. Makes 3 sandwiches.

CHICKPEA SALAD POCKETS: Stuff one-quarter of the chickpea mixture into a pita pocket. Add chopped cucumber, tomato slices, and shredded lettuce. Makes 4 pockets.

PER SERVING: 163 calories; 4 g fat; 0.5 g saturated fat; 22% calories from fat; 0 mg cholesterol; 8 g protein; 25.6 g carbohydrate; 3.5 g sugar; 6.5 g fiber; 525 mg sodium; 72 mg calcium; 2.9 mg iron; 15.2 mg vitamin C; 2555 mcg beta-carotene; 1.2 mg vitamin E

Pan-Seared Portobello Mushrooms

Portobellos are meaty and delicious. They lend themselves well to grilling and can be served on a bed of grains, with mashed potatoes, or on whole-grain buns with all the trimmings. Plus, they don't contain any of the carcinogens that are formed when meat is cooked. Portobello mushrooms are a great source of folate, selenium, and zinc.

4 large portobello mushrooms

2 tablespoons red wine or water

2 tablespoons reduced-sodium soy sauce

1 tablespoon balsamic vinegar

2 garlic cloves, minced or pressed

½ teaspoon dried oregano

1. Clean the mushrooms and trim the stems so they are flush with bottom of the caps.

2. Combine the wine, soy sauce, vinegar, garlic, and oregano in a large skillet. Heat until the mixture begins to bubble. Add the mushrooms, top side down. Lower the heat to medium, cover, and cook for 3 minutes. If the pan becomes dry, add 2 to 3 tablespoons of water. Turn the mushrooms over and cook for about 5 minutes longer, until they are tender when pierced with a sharp knife. Serve hot.

3. Stored in a covered container in the refrigerator, leftover Pan-Seared Portobello Mushrooms will keep for up to 3 days.

PER SERVING: 38 calories; 0.5 g fat; 0 g saturated fat; 12.9% calories from fat; 0 mg cholesterol; 3.3 g protein; 4.9 g total carbohydrate; 0.2 g sugar; 1.8 g fiber; 273 mg sodium; 10 mg calcium; 0.7 mg iron; 0.5 mg vitamin C; 5 mcg beta-carotene; 0 mg vitamin E

Quick Bean Burritos

These burritos wrap up a perfect balance of flavor and nutrition. They are versatile enough that you can add any leftover vegetables, grains, or beans that are in your refrigerator.

1 can (15 ounces) **low-fat vegetarian refried beans**

4 whole wheat tortillas

1 cup shredded romaine lettuce

1 cup Calabacitas (page 175; optional)

½ cup Mango Salsa (page 111) **or other favorite salsa**

½ cup Low-Fat Guacamole (page 110)

2 green onions, chopped

1. Heat the refried beans in small saucepan or in a microwave until warmed through.

2. Warm the tortillas, one at a time, in a dry skillet over medium heat. Alternatively, warm the tortillas in the microwave.

3. Spread one-quarter of the beans down the center of each tortilla and top with the remaining ingredients. Fold the bottom end of each tortilla toward the center, then roll the tortilla around the filling. Alternatively, place all of the ingredients on the table and let everyone assemble their own burritos.

PER SERVING: 208 calories; 3.1 g fat; 0.5 g saturated fat; 13.4% calories from fat; 0 mg cholesterol; 10.1 g protein; 37.9 g carbohydrate; 2.4 g sugar; 9.8 g fiber; 713 mg sodium; 57 mg calcium; 2.8 mg iron; 15.2 mg vitamin C; 637 mcg beta-carotene; 1.2 mg vitamin E

Quinoa Tacos

lthough quinoa is typically used as a grain, it is actually a seed native to South America. It is high in protein and can be used as an alternative to rice.

4 cups water

¼ teaspoon salt

2 cups quinoa, rinsed and drained

3 cups cooked or canned black beans, rinsed and drained

2 garlic cloves, minced or pressed

12 whole wheat tortillas

2 cups Low-Fat Guacamole (page 110)

3 tablespoons chopped fresh cilantro

5 cups chopped romaine lettuce

1 cup salsa

1. Bring the water and salt to a boil in a medium saucepan. Add the quinoa, cover, lower the heat to medium-low, and cook for 20 minutes. Remove from the heat and set aside.

2. Combine the beans and garlic in a shallow pan and warm over medium-low heat for 5 minutes.

3. If desired, warm the tortillas, one at a time, in a dry skillet over medium heat. Alternatively, warm the tortillas in a microwave.

4. Fill the tortillas with the quinoa, beans, guacamole, and cilantro. Top with the lettuce and salsa and serve.

PER SERVING: 358 calories; 7.5 g fat; 1.4 g saturated fat; 18.8% calories from fat; 0 mg cholesterol; 13 g protein; 61.1 g carbohydrate; 4.5 g sugar; 10 g fiber; 1188 mg sodium; 133 mg calcium; 5.9 mg iron; 8.6 mg vitamin C; 791 mcg beta-carotene; 1.3 mg vitamin E

Red Bean Wraps

Instead of buying fast food, prepare these wholesome wraps whenever you need a quick meal. They are delicious hot or cold and are loaded with health-supporting fiber. The chile adds spiciness; you can use more or less according to your taste.

1½ cups cooked or canned red or pinto beans, rinsed and drained

½ cup chopped fresh cilantro

1 Anaheim chile, seeded and finely chopped

1 garlic clove, peeled

½ teaspoon salt

4 whole wheat tortillas

½ cup salsa

½ cup finely chopped sweet onion

1 large tomato, chopped

1 to 2 cups prewashed salad mix

1. Combine the beans, cilantro, chile, garlic, and salt in a food processor and process until smooth.
2. For warm wraps, heat the bean mixture in a microwave. Warm the tortillas, one at a time, in a dry skillet over medium heat. Alternatively, warm the tortillas in the microwave. Spread one-quarter of the bean mixture in a line down the middle of each tortilla. Top with the remaining ingredients in the order listed and roll each tortilla around the filling.

PER SERVING: 209 calories; 1.8 g fat; 0.3 g saturated fat; 7.5% calories from fat; 0 mg cholesterol; 10.9 g protein; 40.6 g carbohydrate; 4.6 g sugar; 9.4 g fiber; 791 mg sodium; 64 mg calcium; 3.3 mg iron; 36.3 mg vitamin C; 899 mcg beta-carotene; 1.1 mg vitamin E

Soft-Shell Tacos

If you enjoy Mexican food, you'll be delighted to learn that a variety of great-tasting meatless taco fillings are available in the refrigerated section of natural food stores and larger supermarkets. If you prefer, you can make your own filling with vegan burger crumbles and Mexican seasonings, as we've done in this recipe.

1 cup water

1 small onion, finely chopped

½ cup finely chopped bell pepper

¼ cup finely chopped fresh cilantro

2 garlic cloves, minced or pressed

4 vegan burger patties (thawed, if frozen), chopped

½ cup tomato sauce or crushed tomatoes

2 to 3 teaspoons chili powder

1 teaspoon ground cumin

¼ teaspoon dried oregano

½ chipotle chile in adobo sauce, finely chopped, or ¼ teaspoon crushed red pepper flakes

8 corn tortillas

½ to 1 cup salsa

3 to 4 green onions, chopped

2 cups shredded romaine lettuce

1 to 2 medium tomatoes, cut into wedges

1 avocado, cut into 8 wedges (optional)

1. Heat ½ cup of the water in a large skillet. Add the onion, bell pepper, cilantro, and garlic. Cook and stir over medium heat for 5 to 10 minutes, until the onion is soft.

2. Add the remaining ½ cup water and the burgers, tomato sauce, chili powder, cumin, oregano, and chile. Stir to mix. Turn the heat to low and cook and stir for 2 to 3 minutes, until the mixture is fairly dry.

3. Warm the tortillas, one at a time, in a dry skillet over medium heat. Flip the tortilla from side to side until soft. Add a spoonful of the filling and fold the tortilla in half over it. Cook for 1 minute on each side. Open the tortilla and add a portion of the remaining ingredients in the order listed. Repeat with remaining tortillas.

PER SERVING: 121 calories; 1.5 g fat; 0.2 g saturated fat; 11.3% calories from fat; 0 mg cholesterol; 8.9 g protein; 21.1 g carbohydrate; 4.1 g sugar; 4.2 g fiber; 371 mg sodium; 104 mg calcium; 2.4 mg iron; 18.9 mg vitamin C; 821 mcg beta-carotene; 1.1 mg vitamin E

Ten-Minute Tostadas

 hese quick tostadas are delicious served with Tex-Mex Bulgur Pilaf (page 170). Vegetarian refried beans are sold in most supermarkets.

1 can (15 ounces) **fat-free vegetarian refried beans**

2 corn tortillas

1 to 2 green onions, sliced

2 cups thinly sliced romaine lettuce or prewashed salad mix

1 medium tomato, chopped

¼ avocado, sliced (optional)

2 teaspoons seasoned rice vinegar

3 tablespoons salsa

1. Heat the refried beans in a small saucepan or in a microwave until very hot.

2. Warm the tortillas, one at a time, in a dry skillet over medium heat. Flip the tortilla from side to side until soft. Transfer to a plate.

3. Spread each tortilla with half of the beans. Top with the green onions, lettuce, tomato, and optional avocado. Sprinkle with the vinegar and salsa.

PER SERVING: 272 calories; 2 g fat; 0.3 g saturated fat; 6.6% calories from fat; 0 mg cholesterol; 14.7 g protein; 52.2 g carbohydrate; 6.5 g sugar; 14.2 g fiber; 1071 mg sodium; 142 mg calcium; 4.1 mg iron; 27.4 mg vitamin C; 2369 mcg beta-carotene; 1.9 mg vitamin E

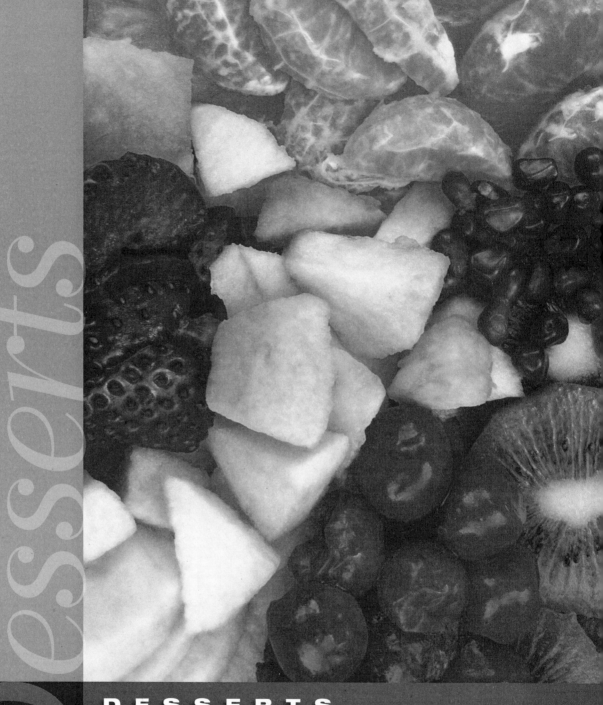

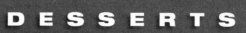

DESSERTS

Ambrosia

This colorful fruit salad may be made up to a day in advance if you add the banana just before serving. Fruit-sweetened desserts not only satisfy a sweet tooth, they're full of health-promoting antioxidants. In this case, you're better off opting *for* dessert!

2 oranges, peeled and chopped

2 cups pineapple chunks

1 banana, sliced

¼ cup unsweetened shredded dried coconut

2 to 4 tablespoons dried cranberries

1 tablespoon orange juice concentrate

1 tablespoon water

½ teaspoon almond extract

1. Combine the oranges, pineapple, banana, coconut, and cranberries in a medium bowl.

2. Combine the orange juice concentrate, water, and almond extract in a small bowl. Pour over the fruit and toss until evenly distributed.

3. Stored in a covered container in the refrigerator, leftover Ambrosia (without the banana) will keep for up to 2 days.

PER SERVING: 188 calories; 2.4 g fat; 1.9 g saturated fat; 11.5% calories from fat; 0 mg cholesterol; 1.8 g protein; 43.3 g carbohydrate; 35.3 g sugar; 3.9 g fiber; 17 mg sodium; 49 mg calcium; 0.7 mg iron; 61.5 mg vitamin C; 88 mcg beta-carotene; 0.3 mg vitamin E

Berry Applesauce

Serve this applesauce hot or cold. Berries give it a deep red or purple color and add a hefty dose of anthocyanins—potent cancer-fighting antioxidants.

2 cups peeled, cored, and diced apples

2 cups fresh or frozen strawberries, blueberries, or raspberries

½ cup frozen apple juice concentrate

1 teaspoon ground cinnamon

1. Combine all of the ingredients in a medium saucepan. Bring to a gentle simmer, cover, and cook over very low heat for about 25 minutes, or until the apples are tender when pierced with a fork. Mash lightly with a potato masher or purée in a food processor, if desired.

2. Stored in a covered container in the refrigerator, leftover Berry Applesauce will keep for up to 3 days.

PER SERVING: 108 calories; 0.4 g fat; 0 g saturated fat; 3.5% calories from fat; 0 mg cholesterol; 0.8 g protein; 26.9 g carbohydrate; 20.1 g sugar; 2.7 g fiber; 11 mg sodium; 29 mg calcium; 0.9 mg iron; 49.2 mg vitamin C; 13 mcg beta-carotene; 0.4 mg vitamin E

Chocolate Mousse or Chocolate Mousse Pie

When consumed in moderation, this is a more healthful version of the traditional high-fat, high-calorie French delicacy. Chocolate contains the phenolic compounds gallic acid and epicatechin, which are important antioxidants for cancer prevention. Cornell researchers have found that cocoa has nearly twice the antioxidants of red wine and up to three times those found in green tea.

1 cup semisweet chocolate chips

1 cup fortified soymilk or other nondairy milk

2 packages (12.3 ounces each) low-fat silken tofu

1 teaspoon vanilla extract

1 (10-inch) ready-made graham cracker pie crust (optional)

10 strawberries, sliced

10 fresh mint sprigs (optional)

1. Place the chocolate chips and soymilk in a microwave-safe bowl and microwave for 1 minute. Let rest for 2 minutes. Alternatively, place the chocolate chips and soymilk in a double boiler over gently simmering water. Heat, stirring occasionally, until the chips are melted.

2. Transfer the chocolate chip mixture to a food processor or blender. Add the tofu and vanilla extract and process until smooth.

3. Pour into the crust, if using, or small individual serving dishes and chill for 2 hours in the refrigerator or 30 minutes in the freezer.

3. Top with the strawberries just before serving and garnish with the optional mint.

4. Stored in a covered container in the refrigerator, leftover Chocolate Mousse or Chocolate Mousse Pie will keep for up to 3 days.

Variation: Add 1 chopped banana to the blender or food processor along with the tofu.

PER SERVING: 125 calories; 6 g fat; 3.1 g saturated fat; 43.5% calories from fat; 0 mg cholesterol; 6 g protein; 14.1 g carbohydrate; 10.5 g sugar; 1.5 g fiber; 75 mg sodium; 63 mg calcium; 1.4 mg iron; 7.2 mg vitamin C; 7 mcg beta-carotene; 0.5 mg vitamin E

Festive Fruited Yams

This recipe contains pectin, a soluble fiber found in fruits and vegetables that can help kill prostate cancer cells. The most concentrated sources of pectin are found in apples, peaches, and citrus fruit. This sweet, low-fat recipe makes an excellent side dish or dessert. Use it is an opportunity to boost your immune system and cancer-fighting capacity over the holiday season.

4 yams or sweet potatoes, peeled and cut into 1-inch pieces

1 large green apple, peeled and sliced

1 cup fresh cranberries, or ¼ cup dried cranberries

½ cup raisins

2 tablespoons sugar or other sweetener

½ cup orange juice

1. Preheat the oven to 350 degrees F.

2. Place the yams in a 9 x 13-inch baking dish. Top with the apple, cranberries, and raisins. Sprinkle with the sugar, and pour the orange juice over all. Cover and bake for 1 hour and 15 minutes, or until the yams are tender when pierced with a fork.

3. Stored in a covered container in the refrigerator, leftover Festive Fruited Yams will keep for up to 3 days.

PER SERVING: 114 calories; 0.2 g fat; 0 g saturated fat; 1.5% calories from fat; 0 mg cholesterol; 1.6 g protein; 28.2 g carbohydrate; 17.6 g sugar; 3.1 g fiber; 23 mg sodium; 33 mg calcium; 0.7 mg iron; 20.1 mg vitamin C; 6571 mcg beta-carotene; 0.6 mg vitamin E

Gingerbread

This gingerbread is simple to prepare and makes a wonderful, low-fat treat. Keeping your fat intake low is crucial for preventing hormone-related cancers, such as breast and prostate cancer, while also allowing your immune system to work at its best. You can use spreadable fruit, thinned with a bit of water, for a scrumptious, fat-free topping.

1¾ cups water

¾ cup sugar

½ cup raisins

2 teaspoons ground cinnamon

1 teaspoon ground ginger

¾ teaspoon ground nutmeg

½ teaspoon salt

¼ teaspoon ground cloves

2 cups all-purpose flour

1 teaspoon baking soda

1 teaspoon baking powder

¼ cup blackstrap molasses

2 tablespoons fortified soymilk or water

1 tablespoon powdered sugar

1. Combine the water, sugar, raisins, cinnamon, ginger, nutmeg, salt, and cloves in a large saucepan and bring to a boil. Boil for 2 minutes. Remove from the heat and let cool completely, either in the refrigerator for 45 minutes or in the freezer for about 15 minutes.

2. Preheat the oven to 350 degrees F. Lightly mist a 9-inch square baking pan with vegetable oil spray.

3. Combine the flour, baking soda, and baking powder in a medium bowl. Gradually stir the flour mixture into the cooled raisin mixture along with the molasses and soymilk. Spread the mixture into the prepared baking pan and bake for 30 minutes, or until a toothpick inserted into the center comes out clean.

4. Sprinkle with the powdered sugar just before slicing.

5. Stored in a covered container, Gingerbread will keep for up to 3 days in the refrigerator or up to 1 month in the freezer.

PER SERVING: 165 calories; 0.4 g fat; 0.1 g saturated fat; 2% calories from fat; 0 mg cholesterol; 2.5 g protein; 38.8 g carbohydrate; 19.6 g sugar; 1.2 g fiber; 211 mg sodium; 92 mg calcium; 2.5 mg iron; 0.3 mg vitamin C; 0 mcg beta-carotene; 0.1 mg vitamin E

Gingered Melon

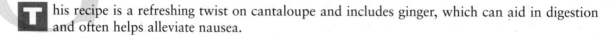

This recipe is a refreshing twist on cantaloupe and includes ginger, which can aid in digestion and often helps alleviate nausea.

1 large cantaloupe

1 tablespoon chopped crystallized ginger

½ teaspoon ground ginger

1. Cut the cantaloupe in half. Scoop out the seeds and cut the flesh into chunks. Sprinkle the crystallized and ground ginger over the cantaloupe and stir. Chill thoroughly before serving.

2. Stored in a covered container in the refrigerator, leftover Gingered Melon will keep for up to 2 days.

Note: To remove the rind from the cantaloupe, place the cut side of the melon on a cutting board. Use a chef's knife or serrated knife to carefully cut off the rind, starting from the top of the melon and working down to the cutting board, rotating the melon as needed. Make sure to secure the melon with your opposite hand and keep your fingers tucked away from the knife's edge.

PER SERVING: 54 calories; 0.3 g fat; 0.1 g saturated fat; 4.6% calories from fat; 0 mg cholesterol; 1.2 g protein; 13.1 g carbohydrate; 12.4 g sugar; 1.3 g fiber; 22 mg sodium; 13 mg calcium; 0.3 mg iron; 49.9 mg vitamin C; 2741 mcg beta-carotene; 0.1 mg vitamin E

Harvest Pudding

 his pudding is quite irresistible when it's hot, so if you want to serve it chilled, make a double batch.

2½ cups fortified soymilk or other nondairy milk

1 cup solid-pack canned pumpkin

½ cup yellow cornmeal

⅓ cup sugar

2 tablespoons light molasses

½ teaspoon ground cinnamon

¼ teaspoon ground ginger

¼ teaspoon salt

1. Combine all of the ingredients in a medium saucepan and whisk until smooth. Bring to a gentle simmer over medium heat and cook, stirring or whisking constantly, for about 15 minutes, until thickened. Spoon into small bowls. Serve warm or chilled.

2. Stored in a covered container in the refrigerator, leftover Harvest Pudding will keep for up to 3 days.

PER SERVING: 173 calories; 2 g fat; 0.3 g saturated fat; 10.3% calories from fat; 0 mg cholesterol; 5 g protein; 35.3 g carbohydrate; 18.4 g sugar; 2.9 g fiber; 199 mg sodium; 163 mg calcium; 2.7 mg iron; 2.1 mg vitamin C; 2846 mcg beta-carotene; 1.8 mg vitamin E

Pumpkin Pie or Custard

Made this way, pumpkin pie can actually be a health food. Pumpkin is a rich source of beta-carotene, a well-known cancer-fighting agent that is also important for cancer survival. Note that the fat in this recipe comes only from the pie crust, so we've provided a nutritional analysis without the crust as well, in case you'd like to serve it as a fat-free baked custard.

1½ cups fortified soymilk

4 tablespoons cornstarch

1½ cups solid-pack canned pumpkin or cooked pumpkin

½ cup sugar

1 teaspoon ground cinnamon

½ teaspoon ground ginger

½ teaspoon salt

⅛ teaspoon ground cloves

1 (9-inch) unbaked pie crust (optional)

1. Preheat the oven to 375 degrees F.

2. Combine the soymilk and cornstarch in a large bowl and whisk until smooth. Stir in the pumpkin, sugar, cinnamon, ginger, salt, and cloves. Pour into the optional pie crust or a custard dish and bake for 45 minutes, or until firm. Cool before slicing the pie or serving the custard.

3. Stored in a covered container in the refrigerator, leftover Pumpkin Pie or Custard will keep for up to 3 days.

PER SERVING (with crust): 185 calories; 6.1 g fat; 1.5 g saturated fat; 29.5% calories from fat; 0 mg cholesterol; 3.2 g protein; 30.6 g total carbohydrate; 14.5 g sugar; 2.4 g fiber; 283 mg sodium; 84 mg calcium; 2 mg iron; 2.2 mg vitamin C; 3189 mcg beta-carotene; 1.2 mg vitamin E

PER SERVING (without crust): 103 calories; 0.9 g fat; 0.2 g saturated fat; 7.9% calories from fat; 0 mg cholesterol; 2.1 g protein; 22.8 g total carbohydrate; 14.5 g sugar; 2.1 g fiber; 181 mg sodium; 83 mg calcium; 1.5 mg iron; 2.2 mg vitamin C; 3189 mcg beta-carotene; 1.1 mg vitamin E

Rice Pudding

J asmine or basmati rice works especially well in this pudding. Serve it as a low-fat treat or dessert; it can even make a great breakfast.

2 cups water

1 cup white rice (preferably jasmine or basmati)

¼ teaspoon salt

1½ cups fortified soymilk or other nondairy milk

⅓ cup maple syrup or agave syrup

2 tablespoons unsweetened shredded dried coconut

½ teaspoon vanilla extract

½ cup golden raisins or chopped dried apricots

1. Combine the water, rice, and salt in a medium saucepan. Cover and simmer over low heat for 15 minutes. Check occasionally and add a small amount of water, if necessary, to prevent sticking.

2. Stir in the soymilk, syrup, coconut, and vanilla extract. Cover and cook over low heat for about 20 minutes, until thickened. Stir in the raisins. Serve warm or thoroughly chilled.

3. Stored in a covered container in the refrigerator, leftover Rice Pudding will keep for up to 3 days.

PER SERVING: 250 calories; 2 g fat; 0.8 g saturated fat; 7.4% calories from fat; 0 mg cholesterol; 5.1 g protein; 53.4 g carbohydrate; 20.1 g sugar; 1.5 g fiber; 142 mg sodium; 103 mg calcium; 2.2 mg iron; 0.5 mg vitamin C; 1 mcg beta-carotene; 0.9 mg vitamin E

Summer Fruit Compote

Although this compote is perfect during summer when peaches and strawberries are in season, it is actually delicious any time of year if frozen fruit is used.

2 cups sliced fresh peaches (peeled, if desired) **or frozen sliced peaches**

2 cups hulled fresh strawberries or frozen strawberries

½ cup white grape juice concentrate or apple juice concentrate

1. Combine all of the ingredients in a large saucepan. Bring to a simmer and cook for about 5 minutes, or until the fruit just becomes soft.

2. Serve warm or thoroughly chilled, by itself or over fruit sorbet or vanilla nondairy ice cream.

3. Stored in a covered container in the refrigerator, leftover Summer Fruit Compote will keep for up to 3 days.

PER SERVING: 121 calories; 0.5 g fat; 0.1 g saturated fat; 4% calories from fat; 0 mg cholesterol; 1.5 g protein; 29.6 g carbohydrate; 26.3 g sugar; 2.8 g fiber; 3 mg sodium; 21 mg calcium; 0.6 mg iron; 77.9 mg vitamin C; 149 mcg beta-carotene; 0.8 mg vitamin E

Tapioca Pudding

Tapioca is a starch derived from the root of the cassava plant. It may be ground into flour for baked goods or used as a thickener in jellies and pie fillings, although its most perfect use may be in this delicious pudding. Using nondairy ingredients is important, since the consumption of dairy foods has been linked to cancers of the prostate, breast, and ovary.

2 cups fortified soymilk or other nondairy milk

¼ cup instant tapioca

¼ cup sugar

¼ teaspoon salt

1 teaspoon vanilla extract

1. Combine the soymilk, tapioca, sugar, and salt in a saucepan and stir to mix. Let stand for 5 minutes.

2. Bring to a boil over medium heat, stirring almost constantly. Remove from the heat and let stand for 15 minutes. The pudding will thicken as it cools. Stir in the vanilla extract. Serve warm or thoroughly chilled.

3. Stored in a covered container in the refrigerator, leftover Tapioca Pudding will keep for up to 3 days.

PER SERVING: 150 calories; 2 g fat; 0.3 g saturated fat; 12% calories from fat; 0 mg cholesterol; 4.3 g protein; 28.9 g carbohydrate; 15.1 g sugar; 1.4 g fiber; 222 mg sodium; 163 mg calcium; 1.6 mg iron; 0.4 mg vitamin C; 1 mcg beta-carotene; 1.7 mg vitamin E

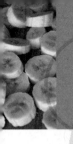

RECIPE CONTRIBUTORS

Stephanie Beine, RD Basic Polenta, Quinoa Pilaf, Raspberry Salad Dressing

Evelisse Capo, PharmD Brown Rice with Black Beans, Grilled Plantains, Latin Seitan Stew, Quinoa Tacos

Amy Lanou, PhD Asian Fusion Salad, Breakfast Home Fries, Calabacitas, Chocolate Mousse or Chocolate Mousse Pie, Citrus Basil Salad, Creamy Spinach Dip, Cucumber, Mango, and Spinach Salad, Low-Fat Guacamole, Mashed Grains and Cauliflower, Mixed Berry Smoothie, Mushroom Gravy, Penne with Kale, Tomatoes, and Olives, Quick Bean Burritos, Spinach Salad with Citrus Fruit, Tomato, Cucumber, and Basil Salad, Veggies in a Blanket, Zippy Yams and Collards

Jennifer Raymond, MS, RD Ambrosia, Applesauce Muffins, Asian Persuasion Coleslaw, Baked Tofu, Baked Tortilla Chips, Balsamic Vinaigrette, Banana-Date Muffins, Banana-Oat Pancakes, Basic White Sauce, Berry Applesauce, Blueberry Smoothie, Braised Kale, Breakfast Scramble, Broccoli à la King, Broccoli or Cauliflower with Sesame Salt, Broccoli Salad, Brown Rice, Brown Rice and Barley, Brown Rice Pilaf, Buckwheat Pasta with Seitan, Bulgur, Bulgur and Orange Salad, Chickpea Burgers, Chickpea Salad Romaine Wraps, Chinese Fried Bulgur, Chunky Ratatouille Sauce, Couscous, Cream of Broccoli Soup, Creamy Dill Dressing, Creamy Root Soup, Eggless Salad Sandwich, Eggplant Lasagne, Festive Fruited Yams, Fiesta Salad, Fruited Breakfast Quinoa, Garlic Mashed Potatoes, Harvest Pudding, Hoppin' John Salad, Hot or Cold Beet Salad, Lentil and Brown Rice Soup, Lentil and Bulgur Salad, Mango Salsa, Miso Soup with Shiitake Mushrooms, Mushroom

Barley Soup, Mushroom Stroganoff over Fettuccine, No-Meat Loaf, Orange Julius, Pan-Seared Portobello Mushrooms, Parsnip Mashed Potatoes, Piquant Dressing, Portuguese Kale and Potato Soup, Potato and Cauliflower Curry, Potato Boats with Spinach Stuffing, Potato Salad, Pumpkin Pie or Custard, Red Bean Wraps, Rice and Carrot Pilaf, Rice Pudding, Rutabaga Mashed Potatoes, Salad of Spicy Greens with Fruit and Pine Nuts, Simple Brown Gravy, Soft-Shell Tacos, Southwest Bean Salad, Soybean Snacks (Edamame), Spinach Salad with Orange, Radicchio, and Sesame, Strawberry Smoothie, Stuffed Mushrooms, Summer Fruit Compote, Sweet Potato Muffins, Sweet-and-Sour Stir-Fry, Sweet-and-Sour Vegetable Stew, Tapioca Pudding, Ten-Minute Tostadas, Texas Caviar, Tex-Mex Bulgur Pilaf, Three Bean Chili, Tofu French Toast, Tomato Soup with White Beans, Tropical Freeze

Jennifer Reilly, RD Any Veggie Coconut Curry, Black Bean Dip, Colorful Corn Salsa, Easy Bean Salad, Gingerbread, Gingered Melon, Green Goodie Smoothie, Green Tea Smoothie, Lazy Lasagne, Lentil Artichoke Stew, Roasted Red Pepper Hummus, Simple Marinara, White Bean Spread with Sun-Dried Tomatoes

Brandi Redo Black Bean Chili, Spaghetti Squash with Sauce, Tempeh Broccoli Sauté

Brie Turner-McGrievy, MS, RD Collard Greens with Almonds, Curried Sweet Potato Soup, Easy Stir-Fry, Home-Style Squash and Pinto Beans, Red Bean Casserole, Roasted Sweet Potato Wedges, Spicy Black Beans and Tomatoes, Sure-Fire Roasted Vegetables

REFERENCES

CHAPTER 1
Fueling Up on Low-Fat Foods

1. Miller K. Estrogen and DNA damage: the silent source of breast cancer? *J Natl Cancer Inst.* 2003;95:100-102.

2. Prentice R, Thompson D, Clifford C, Gorbach S, Goldin B, Byar D. Dietary fat reduction and plasma estradiol concentration in healthy postmenopausal women. The Women's Health Trial Study Group. *J Natl Cancer Inst.* 1990;82:129-134.

3. Heber D, Ashley JM, Leaf DA, Barnard RJ. Reduction of serum estradiol in postmenopausal women given free access to low-fat high-carbohydrate diet. *Nutrition.* 1991;7:137-139.

4. Dorgan JF, Hunsberger SA, McMahon RP, et al. Diet and sex hormones in girls: findings from a randomized controlled clinical trial. *J Natl Cancer Inst.* 2003;95:132-141.

5. Prentice RL, Caan B, Chlebowski RT, et al. Low-fat dietary pattern and risk of invasive breast cancer: the Women's Health Initiative Randomized Controlled Dietary Modification Trial. *JAMA.* 2006;295:629-642.

6. Gregorio DI, Emrich LJ, Graham S, Marshall JR, Nemoto T. Dietary fat consumption and survival among women with breast cancer. *J Natl Cancer Inst.* 1985 Jul;75(1):37-41.

7. Chlebowski RT. Dietary fat reduction in post-menopausal women with primary breast cancer: Phase III Women's Intervention Nutrition Study (WINS). Paper presented at: American Society of Clinical Oncology Annual Meeting; May 16, 2005; Torrance, CA.

8. Fradet Y, Meyer F, Bairati I, Shadmani R. Dietary fat and prostate cancer progression and survival. *Eur Urol.* 1999;388:91.

9. Saxe GA, Hebert JR, Carmody JF, et al. Can diet in conjunction with stress reduction affect the rate of increase in prostate specific antigen after biochemical recurrence of prostate cancer? *J Urol.* 2001;266:2202-2207.

10. Tymchuk CN, Barnard RJ, Ngo TH, Aronson WJ. Role of testosterone, estradiol, and insulin in diet- and exercise-induced reductions in serum-stimulated prostate cancer cell growth in vitro. *Nutr Cancer.* 2002;42:112-116.

11. Tymchuk CN, Barnard RJ, Heber D, Aronson WJ. Evidence of an inhibitory effect of diet and exercise on prostate cancer cell growth. *J Urol.* 2001;166: 1185-1189.

CHAPTER 3
Discovering Dairy Alternatives

1. Giovannucci E, Rimm EB, Wolk A, et al. Calcium and fructose intake in relation to risk of prostate cancer. *Cancer Res.* 1998;58:442-447.

2. Chan JM, Stampfer MJ, Ma J, Gann PH, Gaziano JM, Giovannucci E. Dairy products, calcium, and prostate cancer risk in the Physicians' Health Study. *Am J Clin Nutr.* 2001;74:549-554.

3. Cadogan J, Eastell R, Jones N, Barker ME. Milk intake and bone mineral acquisition in adolescent girls: randomised, controlled intervention trial. *BMJ.* 1997;315:1255-1260.

4. Heaney RP, McCarron DA, Dawson-Hughes B, et al. Dietary changes favorably affect bone remodeling in older adults. *J Am Dietetic Assoc.* 1999;99: 1228-1233.

5. Cohen P. Serum insulin-like growth factor-I levels and prostate cancer risk—interpreting the evidence. *J Natl Cancer Inst.* 1998;90:876-879.

6. Hankinson SE, Willett WC, Colditz GA, et al. Circulating concentrations of insulin-like growth factor-I and risk of breast cancer. *Lancet.* 1998; 351:1393-1396.

7. Qin LQ, Xu JY, Wang PY, Kaneko T, Hoshi K, Sato A. Milk consumption is a risk factor for prostate cancer: meta-analysis of case-control studies. *Nutr Cancer.* 2004;48(1):22-27.

8. Gao X, LaValley MP, Tucker KL. Prospective studies of dairy product and calcium intakes and prostate cancer risk: a meta-analysis. *J Natl Cancer Inst.* 2005 Dec 7;97(23):1768-1777.

9. Larsson SC, Orsini N, Wolk A. Milk, milk products and lactose intake and ovarian cancer risk: a

meta-analysis of epidemiological studies. *Int J Cancer.* 2006 Jan 15;118(2):431-441.

10. Peyrat JP, Bonneterre J, Hecquet B, et al. Plasma insulin-like growth factor-1 (IGF-1) concentrations in human breast cancer. *Eur J Cancer.* 1993;29A: 492-497.

11. Lloyd T, Chinchilli VM, Johnson-Rollings N, Kieselhorst K, Eggli DF, Marcus R. Adult female hip bone density reflects teenage sports-exercise patterns but not teenage calcium intake. *Pediatrics.* 2000;106:40-44.

12. Feskanich D, Willett WC, Colditz GA. Calcium, vitamin D, milk consumption, and hip fractures: a prospective study among postmenopausal women. *Am J Clin Nutr.* 2003;77:504-511.

CHAPTER 4
Replacing Meat

1. Thorogood M, Mann J, Appleby P, McPherson K. Risk of death from cancer and ischaemic heart disease in meat and non-meat eaters. *Br Med J.* 1994;308:1667-1670.

2. Chang-Claude J, Frentzel-Beyme R, Eilber U. Mortality patterns of German vegetarians after 11 years of follow-up. *Epidemiol.* 1992;3:395-401.

3. Chang-Claude J, Frentzel-Beyme R. Dietary and lifestyle determinants of mortality among German vegetarians. *Int J Epidemiol.* 1993;22:228-236.

4. Barnard ND, Nicholson A, Howard JL. The medical costs attributable to meat consumption. *Prev Med.* 1995;24:646-655.

5. Willett WC, Stampfer MJ, Colditz GA, Rosner BA, Speizer FE. Relation of meat, fat, and fiber intake to the risk of colon cancer in a prospective study among women. *N Engl J Med.* 1990;323: 1664-1672.

6. Giovannucci E, Rimm EB, Stampfer MJ, Colditz GA, Ascherio A, Willett WC. Intake of fat, meat, and fiber in relation to risk of colon cancer in men. *Cancer Res.* 1994;54:2390-2397.

7. Chao A, Thun MJ, Connell CJ, et al. Meat consumption and risk of colorectal cancer. *JAMA.* 2005;293:172-182.

8. Fraser GE. Associations between diet and cancer, ischemic heart disease, and all-cause mortality in non-Hispanic white California Seventh-day Adventists. *Am J Clin Nutr.* 1999;70(suppl):532S-538S.

9. Meyerhardt JA, Niedzwecki D, Hollis D, et al. Association of dietary pattern with cancer recurrence and survival in patients with stage III colon cancer. *JAMA.* 2007;298:754-764.

10. Lewin MH, Bailey N, Bandaletova T, et al. Red meat enhances the colonic formation of the DNA adduct O^6-carboxylmethyl guanine: implications for colorectal cancer. *Cancer Res.* 2006;66: 1859-1865.

11. Sinha R, Rothman N, Brown ED, et al. High concentrations of the carcinogen 2-amino-1-methyl-6-phenylimidazo-[4,5] pyridine [PhIP] occur in chicken but are dependent on the cooking method. *Cancer Res.* 1995;55:4516-4519.

12. American Dietetic Association, Dietitians of Canada. Position of the American Dietetic Association and Dietitians of Canada: vegetarian diets. *J Am Diet Assoc.* 2003 Jun;103(6):748-765.

CHAPTER 5
Cancer-Fighting Compounds and Immune-Boosting Foods

1. Rock CL, Demark-Wahnefried W. Nutrition and survival after the diagnosis of breast cancer: a review of the evidence. *J Clin Oncol.* 2002;20:3302-3316.

2. Murillo G, Mehta RG. Cruciferous vegetables and cancer prevention. *Nutr Cancer.* 2001;41:17-28.

3. Bendich A. Carotenoids and the immune response. *J Nut.* 1989;119:112-115.

4. Watson RR, Prabhala RH, Plezia PM, Alberts DS. Effect of beta-carotene on lymphocyte subpopulations in elderly humans: evidence for a dose-response relationship. *Am J Clin Nutr.* 1991; 53:90-94.

5. Institute of Medicine. Food and Nutrition Board. Dietary reference intakes for vitamin A, vitamin K, arsenic, boron, chromium, copper, iodine, iron, manganese, molybdenum, nickel, silicon, vanadium, and zinc. National Academy Press, Washington, DC, 2001.

6. Giovannucci E, Rimm EB, Liu Y, Stampfer MJ, Willett WC. A prospective study of tomato products, lycopene, and prostate cancer risk. *J Natl Cancer Inst.* 2002;94:391-398.

7. Saintot M, Matthieu-Daude H, Astre C, Grenier J, Simony-Lafontaine J, Gerber M. Oxidant-antioxidant status in relation to survival among breast cancer patients. *Int J Cancer.* 2002;97:574-579.

8. Chandra RK. Nutrition and the immune system from birth to old age. *Eur J Clin Nutr.* 2002;56: S73-S76.

9. Kensler TW, Chen JG, Egner PA, et al. Effects of glucosinolate-rich broccoli sprouts on urinary levels of aflatoxin-DNA adducts and phenanthrene tetraols in a randomized clinical trial in He Zuo township, Qidong, People's Republic of China. *Cancer Epidemiol Biomarkers Prev.* 2005 Nov; 14(11 Pt 1):2605-2613.

10. Chiao JW, Chung FL, Kancherla R, Ahmed T, Mittelman A, Conaway CC. Sulforaphane and its metabolite mediate growth arrest and apoptosis in human prostate cancer cells. *Int J Oncol.* 2002;20:631-636.

11. Bell MC, Crowley-Nowick P, Bradlow HL, et al. Placebo-controlled trial of indole-3-carbinol in the treatment of CIN. *Gynecol Oncol.* 2000; 78:123-129.

12. Le Bon AM, Siess MH. Organosulfur compounds from *Allium* and their chemoprevention of cancer. *Drug Metabol Drug Interact.* 2000;17:51-79.

13. Pinto JT, Lapsia S, Shah A, Santiago H, Kim G. Antiproliferative effects of garlic-derived and other allium related compounds. *Adv Exp Med Biol.* 2001;492:83-106.

14. Nagourney RA. Garlic: medicinal food or nutritious medicine. *J Medicinal Food.* 1998;1:13-28.

15. Song K, Milner JA. The influence of heating on the anticancer properties of garlic. *J Nutr.* 2001; 131:1054S-1057S.

16. Adom KK, Liu RH. Antioxidant activity of grains *J Agric. Food Chem.* 2002;50:6182-6187.

17. Dardenne M. Zinc and immune function. *Eur J Clin Nutr.* 2002;56:S20-S23.

18. Bogden JD, Oleske JM, Lavenhar MA, et al. Effects of one year of supplementation with zinc and other micronutrients on cellular immunity in the elderly. *J Am Coll Nutr.* 1990;9:214-225.

19. Hawley HP, Gordon GB. The effects of long chain free fatty acids on human neutrophil function and structure. *Lab Invest.* 1976;34:216-222.

20. Nordenstrom J, Jarstrand C, Wiernik A. Decreased chemotactic and random migration of leukocytes during intralipid infusion. *Am J Clin Nutr.* 1979; 32:2416-2422.

21. Von Schacky CS, Fischer S, Weber PC. Long-term effect of dietary marine omega-3 fatty acids upon plasma and cellular lipids, platelet function, and eicosanoid formation in humans. *J Clin Invest.* 1985;76:1626-1631.

22. Endres S, Ghorbani R, Kelley VE, et al. The effect of dietary supplementation with n-3 polyunsaturated fatty acids on the synthesis of interleukin-1 and tumor necrosis factor by mononuclear cells. *N Engl J Med.* 1989;320:265-271.

23. Lamas O, Marti A, Martinez JA. Obesity and immunocompetence. *Eur J Clin Nutr.* 2002; 56:S42-S45.

24. Malter M, Schriever G, Eilber U. Natural killer cells, vitamins, and other blood components of vegetarian and omnivorous men. *Nutr Cancer.* 1989;12:271-278.

CHAPTER 6
Maintaining a Healthy Weight

1. Rock CL, Demark-Wahnefried W. Nutrition and survival after the diagnosis of breast cancer: a review of the evidence. *J Clin Oncol.* 2002; 20:3302-3316.

2. Lamas O, Marti A, Martinez JA. Obesity and immunocompetence. *Eur J Clin Nutr.* 2002;56 (Suppl 1):S42-S45.

3. Howarth NC, Saltzman E, Roberts SB. Dietary fiber and weight regulation. *Nutr Rev.* 2001; 59:129-139.

4. Barnard ND, Scialli AR, Turner-McGrevy G, Lanou AJ, Glass J. The effects of a low-fat plant-based dietary intervention on body weight, metabolism, and insulin sensitivity. *Am J Med.* 2005; 118:991-997.

5. Barnard ND, Scialli AR, Hurlock D, Bertron P. Diet and sex-hormone binding globulin, dysmenorrhea, and premenstrual symptoms. *Obstet Gynecol.* 2000;95:245-250.

6. Barnard ND, Cohen J, Jenkins DJ, et al. A low-fat vegan diet improves glycemic control and cardiovascular risk factors in a randomized clinical trial in individuals with type 2 diabetes. *Diabetes Care.* 2006 Aug;29(8):1777-1783.

7. Berkow SE, Barnard N. Vegetarian diets and weight status. *Nutr Rev.* 2006 Apr;64(4):175-188.

8. Reddy ST, Wang CY, Sakhaee K, Brinkley L, Pak CY. Effect of low-carbohydrate high-protein diets on acid-base balance, stone-forming propensity, and calcium metabolism. *Am J Kidney Dis.* 2002; 40:265-274.

9. Willett WC, Stampfer MJ, Colditz GA, Rosner BA, Speizer FE. Relation of meat, fat, and fiber

intake to the risk of colon cancer in a prospective study among women. *N Engl J Med.* 1990;323:1664-1672.

10. Giovannucci E, Rimm EB, Stampfer MJ, Colditz GA, Ascherio A, Willett WC. Intake of fat, meat, and fiber in relation to risk of colon cancer in men. *Cancer Res.* 1994;54:2390-2397.

CHAPTER 7
Foods and Breast Cancer Survival

1. Wynder EL, Kajitani T, Kuno J, Lucas JC Jr, DePalo A, Farrow J. A comparison of survival rates between American and Japanese patients with breast cancer. *Surg Gynecol Obstet.* 1963;117:196-200.

2. Rock CL, Demark-Wahnefried W. Nutrition and survival after the diagnosis of breast cancer: a review of the evidence. *J Clin Oncol.* 2002;20:3302-3316.

3. Tao MH, Shu XO, Ruan ZX, Gao YT, Zheng W. Association of overweight with breast cancer survival. *Am J Epidemiol.* 2006;163:101-107.

4. Verreault R, Brisson J, Deschenes L, Naud F, Meyer F, Belanger L. Dietary fat in relation to prognostic indicators in breast cancer. *J Natl Cancer Inst.* 1988;80:819-825.

5. Hebert JR, Toporoff E. Dietary exposures and other factors of possible prognostic significance in relation to tumour size and nodal involvement in early-stage breast cancer. *Int J Epidemiol.* 1989;18:518-526.

6. Gregorio DI, Emrich LJ, Graham S, Marshall JR, Nemoto T. Dietary fat consumption and survival among women with breast cancer. *J Natl Cancer Inst.* 1985 Jul;75(1):37-41.

7. Nomura A, Le Marchand L, Kolonel LN, Hankin JH. The effect of dietary fat on breast cancer survival among Caucasian and Japanese women in Hawaii. *Breast Cancer Res and Treatment.* 1991;18:S135-S141.

8. Holm LE, Nordevang E, Hjalmar ML, Lidbrink E, Callmer E, Nilsson B. Treatment failure and dietary habits in women with breast cancer. *J Natl Cancer Inst.* 1993;85:32-36.

9. Jain M, Miller AB, To T. Premorbid diet and the prognosis of women with breast cancer. *J Natl Cancer Inst.* 1994;86:1390-1397.

10. Zhang S, Folsom AR, Sellers TA, Kushi LH, Potter JD. Better breast cancer survival for post-menopausal women who are less overweight and eat less fat. *Cancer.* 1995;76:275-283.

11. Rohan TE, Hiller JE, McMichael AJ. Dietary factors and survival from breast cancer. *Nutr Cancer.* 1993;20:167-177.

12. Kyogoku S, Hirohata T, Nomura Y, Shigematsu T, Takeshita S, Hirohata I. Diet and prognosis of breast cancer. *Nutr Cancer.* 1992:17:271-277.

13. Newman SC, Miller AB, Howe GR. A study of the effect of weight and dietary fat on breast cancer survival time. *Am J Epidemiol.* 1986;123:767-774.

14. Ewertz M, Gillanders S, Meyer L, Zedeler K. Survival of breast cancer patients in relation to factors which affect risk of developing breast cancer. *Int J Cancer.* 1991;49:526-530.

15. Chlebowski RT, Blackburn GL, Thomson CA, et al. Dietary fat reduction and breast cancer outcome: interim efficacy results from the Women's Intervention Nutrition Study. *J Natl Cancer Inst.* 2006;98:1767-1776.

16. Prentice RI, Caan B, Chlebowski RT, et al. Low-fat dietary pattern and risk of invasive breast cancer: the Women's Health Initiative Randomized Controlled Dietary Modification Trial. *JAMA.* 2006;295:629-642.

17. Holm LE, Callmer E, Hjalmar ML, Lidbrink E, Nilsson B, Skoog L. Dietary habits and prognostic factors in breast cancer. *J Natl Cancer Inst.* 1989;81:1218-1223.

18. Murillo G, Mehta RG. Cruciferous vegetables and cancer prevention. *Nutr Cancer.* 2001;41:17-28.

19. Ingram D. Diet and subsequent survival in women with breast cancer. *Br J Cancer.* 1994;69:592-595.

20. Tartter PI, Papatestas AE, Ioannovich J, Mulvihill MN, Lesnick G, Aufses AH. Cholesterol and obesity as prognostic factors in breast cancer. *Cancer.* 1981;47:2222-2227.

21. Pierce JP, Faerber S, Wright FA, et al. A randomized trial of the effect of a plant-based dietary pattern on additional breast cancer events and survival: the Women's Healthy Eating and Living (WHEL) Study. *Contr Clin Trials.* 2002;23:728-756.

22. Rock CL, Flatt SW, Thomson CA, et al. Effects of a high-fiber, low-fat diet intervention on serum concentrations of reproductive steroid hormones in women with a history of breast cancer. *J Clin Oncol.* 2004;12:2379-2387.

23. Rock CL, Flatt SW, Natarajan L, et al. Plasma carotenoids and recurrence-free survival in women with a history of breast cancer. *J Clin Oncol.* 2005; 23:6631-6638.

24. Pierce JP, Stefanick ML, Flatt SW, et al. Greater survival after breast cancer in physically active women with high vegetable-fruit intake regardless of obesity. *J Clin Oncol.* 2007;25:2345-2351.

25. Pierce JP, Natarajan L, Caan BJ, et al. Influence of a diet very high in vegetables, fruit, and fiber and low in fat on prognosis following treatment for breast cancer: the Women's Healthy Eating and Living (WHEL) randomized trial. *JAMA.* 2007; 298:289-298.

26. Holmes MD, Chen WY, Feskanich D, Kroenke CH, Colditz GA. Physical activity and survival after breast cancer diagnosis. *JAMA.* 2005 May 25; 293(20):2479-2486.

CHAPTER 8
Foods and Prostate Cancer Survival

1. Breslow N, Chan CW, Dhom G, et al. Latent carcinoma of prostate at autopsy in seven areas. *Int J Cancer.* 1977;20:680-688.

2. Fradet Y, Meyer F, Bairati I, Shadmani R. Dietary fat and prostate cancer progression and survival. *Eur Urol.* 1999;388:91.

3. Kim DJ, Gallagher RP, Hislop TG, et al. Premorbid diet in relation to survival from prostate cancer (Canada). *Cancer Causes and Control.* 2000; 11:65-77.

4. Ornish D, Weidner G, Fair WR, et al. Intensive lifestyle changes may affect the progression of prostate cancer. *J Urol.* 2005 Sep;174(3):1065-1070.

5. Carter JP, Saxe GP, Newbold V, Peres CE, Campeau RJ, Bernal-Green L. Hypothesis: dietary management may improve survival from nutritionally linked cancers based on analysis of representative cases. *J Am Coll Nutr.* 1993;12:209-226.

6. Saxe GA, Hebert JR, Carmody JF, et al. Can diet in conjunction with stress reduction affect the rate of increase in prostate specific antigen after biochemical recurrence of prostate cancer? *J Urol.* 2001;266:2202-2207.

7. Tymchuk CN, Barnard RJ, Ngo TH, Aronson WJ. Role of testosterone, estradiol, and insulin in diet- and exercise-induced reductions in serum-stimulated prostate cancer cell growth in vitro. *Nutr Cancer.* 2002;42:112-116.

8. Tymchuk CN, Barnard RJ, Heber D, Aronson WJ. Evidence of an inhibitory effect of diet and exercise on prostate cancer cell growth. *J Urol.* 2001;166: 1185-1189.

9. Giovannucci E, Ascherio A, Rimm EB, et al. Intake of carotenoids and retinol in relation to risk of prostate cancer. *J Natl Cancer Inst.* 1995 Dec 6;87(23):1767-1776.

10. Giovannucci E, Rimm EB, Liu Y, et al. A prospective study of tomato products, lycopene, and prostate cancer risk. *J Natl Cancer Inst.* 2002; 94:391-398.

11. Etminan M, Takkouche B, Caamano-Isorna F. The role of tomato products and lycopene in the prevention of prostate cancer: a meta-analysis of observational studies. *Cancer Epidemiol Biomarkers Prev.* 2004;13:340-345.

12. Kucuk O, Sarkar FH, Djuric Z, et al. Effects of lycopene supplementation in patients with localized prostate cancer. *Exp Biol Med.* 2002;227: 881-885.

CHAPTER 10
Questions and Answers about Foods and Cancer Prevention and Survival

1. Smith-Warner SA, Spiegelman D, Yaun SS, et al. Alcohol and breast cancer in women: a pooled analysis of cohort studies. *JAMA.* 1998; 279(7): 535-540.

2. Boffetta P, Hashibe M. Alcohol and cancer. *Lancet Oncol.* 2006;72:149-156.

3. Tavani A, La Vecchia C. Coffee and cancer: a review of epidemiological studies, 1990-1999. *Eur J Cancer Prev.* 2000;9(4):241-256. Review.

4. Chow WH, Swanson CA, Lissowska J, et al. Risk of stomach cancer in relation to consumption of cigarettes, alcohol, tea and coffee in Warsaw, Poland. *Int J Cancer.* 1999; 81(6):871-876.

5. Tavani A, La Vecchia C. Coffee and cancer: a review of epidemiological studies, 1990-1999. *Eur J Cancer Prev.* 2000;9(4):241-256. Review.

6. World Cancer Research Fund. Food, nutrition and the prevention of cancer: a global perspective. WCRF-AICR, Washington, DC, 2007.

7. Qin LQ, Xu JY, Wang PY, Kaneko T, Hoshi K, Sato A. Milk consumption is a risk factor for prostate cancer: meta-analysis of case-control studies. *Nutr Cancer.* 2004;48(1):22-27.

8. Cohen P. Serum insulin-like growth factor-1 levels and prostate cancer risk—interpreting the evidence. *J Natl Cancer Inst.* 1998;90:876-879.

9. Frazier AL, Ryan CT, Rockett H, Willett WC, Colditz GA. Adolescent diet and risk of breast cancer. *Breast Cancer Res.* 2003;5(3):R59-R64.

10. Stoll BA. Western diet, early puberty, and breast cancer risk. *Breast Cancer Res Treat.* 1998;49(3): 187-193.

11. Link LB, Potter JD. Raw versus cooked vegetables and cancer risk. *Cancer Epidemiol Biomarkers and Prev.* 2004;13(9):1422-1435.

12. The Environmental Working Group. Canaries in the kitchen: teflon toxicosis: DuPont has known for 50 years. http://www.ewg.org/node/8302.

13. Washburn ST, Binman TS, Braithwaite SK, et al. Exposure assessment and risk characterization for perfluorooctanoate in selected consumer articles. *Environ Sci Technol.* 2005;39(11):3904-3910.

14. Darbre PD. Aluminium, antiperspirants and breast cancer. *J Inorg Biochem.* 2005;99(9):1912-1919.

15. Prentice RL, Caan B, Chlebowski RT, et al. Low-fat dietary pattern and risk of invasive breast cancer: the Women's Health Initiative Randomized Controlled Dietary Modification Trial. *JAMA.* 2006;295:629-642.

16. Fradet Y, Meyer F, Bairati I, Shadmani R. Dietary fat and prostate cancer progression and survival. *Eur Urol.* 1999;35:388-391.

17. Hunter JE. n-3 fatty acids from vegetable oils. *Am J Clin Nutr.* 1990;51:809-814.

18. Fraser GE. Risk factors for all-cause and coronary heart disease and mortality in the oldest old. The Adventist Health Study. *Arch Intern Med.* 1999; 53(8):585-590.

19. Zhang J, Zhao Z, Berkel HJ. Egg consumption and mortality from colon and rectal cancers: an ecological study. *Nutr Cancer.* 2003;46(2):158-165.

20. Iscovich JM, L'Abbe KA, Castelleto R. Colon cancer in Argentina. I: risk from intake of dietary items. *Int J Cancer.* 1992;51(6):851-857.

21. Radosavljevic V, Jankovic S, Marinkovic J, Dokic M. Diet and bladder cancer: a case-control study. *Int Urol Nephrol.* 2005;37(2):283-289.

22. London SJ, Yuan JM, Chung FL, et al. Isothiocyanates, glutathione S-transferase M1 and T1 polymorphisms, and lung-cancer risk: a prospective study of men in Shanghai, China. *Lancet.* 2000;356(9231):724-729.

23. Kushi LH, Cunningham JE, Herbert JR, Lerman RH, Bandera EV, Teas J. The macrobiotic diet in cancer. *J Nutr.* 2001;131(11 Suppl):3056S-3064S.

24. The Environmental Working Group. Shoppers guide to pesticides in produce. Retrieved March 12, 2007, at http://www.foodnews.org/.

25. U.S. Department of Health and Human Services, Public Health Service, National Toxicology Program. 2005. 11th report on carcinogens. Available at http://ntp.niehs.nih.gov/ntp/roc/toc11.html.

26. Lee JK, Park BJ, Yoo KY, Ahn YO. Dietary factors and stomach cancer: a case-control study in Korea. *Int J Epidemiol.* 1995;24(1):33-41.

27. Brzezinski A, Debi A. Phytoestrogens: the "natural" selective estrogen receptor modulators? *Eur J Obstet Gynecol Reprod Biol.* 1999;85:47-51.

28. Kurzer MS. Hormonal effects of soy in premenopausal women and men. *J Nutr.* 2002; 132:570S-573S.

29. Messina M, Barnes S. The role of soy products in reducing risk of cancer. *J Natl Cancer Inst.* 1991; 83:541-546.

30. Strom BL, Schinnar R, Ziegler EE, et al. Exposure to soy-based formula in infancy and endocrinological and reproductive outcomes in young adulthood. *JAMA.* 2001;286(7):807-814.

31. Krone CA, Ely JT. Controlling hyperglycemia as an adjunct to cancer therapy. *Integr Cancer Ther.* 2005;4(1):25-31.

32. Michaud DS, Lin S, Giovanucci E, Willet WC, Colditz GA, Fuchs CS. Dietary sugar, glycemic load, and pancreatic cancer risk in a prospective study. *J Natl Cancer Inst.* 2002;94(17):1293-1300.

33. Dufresne CJ, Farnworth ER. A review of latest research findings on the health promotion properties of tea. *J Nutri Biochem.* 2001;12(7):404-421.

34. Kuriyama S, Shimazu T, Ohmori K, et al. Green tea consumption and mortality due to cardiovascular disease, cancer, and all causes in Japan: the Ohsaki study. *JAMA.* 2006;296(10):1255-1265.

35. Graham HN. Green tea composition, consumption, and polyphenol chemistry. *Prev Med.* 1992;21(3):334-350.

ADDITIONAL RESOURCES

NUTRITION INFORMATION

Barnard, Neal. *Food for Life*, Harmony Books, 1993.

———. *Eat Right, Live Longer*, Harmony Books, 1995.

———. *Foods That Fight Pain*, Harmony Books, 1998.

———. *Turn Off the Fat Genes*, Harmony Books, 2001.

———. *Dr. Neal Barnard's Program for Reversing Diabetes*, Rodale Press, 2007.

Davis, Brenda, and Vesanto, Melina. *Becoming Vegan*, Book Publishing Company, 2000.

McDougall, John. *The McDougall Program*, Plume Books, 1991.

Moran, Victoria. *The Love-Powered Diet*, New World Library, 1992.

Ornish, Dean. *Dr. Dean Ornish's Program for Reversing Heart Disease*, Random House, 1990.

———. *Eat More, Weigh Less*, HarperCollins, 1993.

Physicians Committee for Responsible Medicine with Vesanto Melina. *Healthy Eating for Life to Prevent and Treat Cancer*, John Wiley & Sons, 2002.

Stepaniak, Jo. *The Vegan Sourcebook*, McGraw-Hill, 2000.

World Cancer Research Fund and American Institute for Cancer Research. *Food, Nutrition, and the Prevention of Cancer: A Global Perspective*, American Institute for Cancer Research, 1997.

World Cancer Research Fund and American Institute for Cancer Research. *Food, Nutrition, and the Prevention of Cancer: A Global Perspective*, American Institute for Cancer Research, 2007.

COOKBOOKS

Barnard, Neal, ed. *The Best in the World*, Physicians Committee for Responsible Medicine, 1998.

Barnard, Tanya, and Sarah Kramer. *How It All Vegan!* Arsenal Pulp Press, 1999.

Bennett, Jannequin. *Very Vegetarian*, Rutledge Hill Press, 2001.

Bronfman, David, and Rachelle Bronfman. *CalciYum!*, Bromedia, 1998.

Davis, Brenda, Bryanna Clark Grogan, and Jo Stepaniak. *Dairy-Free and Delicious*, Book Publishing Company, 2001.

Keller, Jennifer, ed., and Neal Barnard. *The Best in the World II*, Physicians Committee for Responsible Medicine, 2002.

Kornfeld, Myra. *The Voluptuous Vegan*, Clarkson N. Potter, 2000.

McDougall, Mary, and John McDougall. *The McDougall Quick & Easy Cookbook*, Plume, 1999.

Oser, Marie. *The Enlightened Kitchen*. John Wiley & Sons, 2002.

Raymond, Jennifer. *Fat-Free & Easy*, Heart & Soul Publications, 1997.

Sass, Lorna. *Lorna Sass' Complete Vegetarian Kitchen*, HarperCollins, 1995.

Stepaniak, Jo. *Table for Two*, Book Publishing Company, 1996.

Stepaniak, Jo. *The Ultimate Uncheese Cookbook*, Book Publishing Co., 2003.

Stepaniak, Jo. *Vegan Deli*, Book Publishing Company, 2001.

DVDS AND VIDEOTAPES

"Dairy Products, Calcium, and Prostate Cancer: A Review of the Evidence" by Edward Giovannucci, MD, ScD. (DVD from The Cancer Project's Nutrition & Cancer Video Series)

"Food for Life" (2 discs, 4 hr., 32 min., 39 sec.; lectures with cooking demonstrations), The Cancer Project

Show 1 (24 min., 34 sec.): "How Foods Fight Cancer"

Show 2 (22 min., 10 sec.): "Fueling Up on Low-Fat Foods"

Show 3 (33 min., 29 sec.): "Favoring Fiber"

Show 4 (34 min., 28 sec.): "Discussing Dairy Alternatives"

Show 5 (28 min., 14 sec.): "Replacing Meat"

Show 6 (35 min., 46 sec.): "Cancer-Fighting Compounds and Immune-Boosting Foods"

Show 7 (30 min., 39 sec.): "Maintaining a Healthy Weight"

Show 8 (36 min., 55 sec.): "Foods and Breast Cancer Survival"

Show 9 (26 min., 24 sec.): "Foods and Prostate Cancer Survival"

"Foods for Cancer Prevention and Survival" (videotape, 45 minutes) by Neal Barnard, MD (from Physicians Committee for Responsible Medicine)

"Protection Against Cancer and Chronic Degenerative Diseases: Plants, Genes, and Enzymes" by Paul Talalay, MD (DVD from The Cancer Project's Nutrition & Cancer Video Series)

"Nutrition and Breast Cancer Survival" by Neal Barnard, MD (DVD from The Cancer Project's Nutrition & Cancer Video Series)

"Keys to Keeping the Change" by Paulette Chandler, MD, MPH. (DVD from The Cancer Project's Nutrition & Cancer Video Series)

"Effects of a Plant-based Diet on Disease Progression in Recurrent Prostate Cancer" by Gordon Saxe, MD, PhD, MPH. (DVD from The Cancer Project's Nutrition & Cancer Video Series)

"Dietary Risk Factors for Pancreatic Cancer" by June M. Chan, ScD. (DVD from The Cancer Project's Nutrition & Cancer Video Series)

"The Evolution of Epidemiologic Knowledge on Food, Nutrition and Cancer, " Lawrence Kushi, ScD. (DVD from The Cancer Project's Nutrition & Cancer Video Series)

"Diet: A Prescription That Works for Long-Term Health and Weight Control," Neal Barnard, MD (DVD from The Cancer Project's Nutrition & Cancer Video Series)

"A Low-Fat, Plant-Based Diet Intervention Can Slow or Stop the Progression of Cancer, " John McDougall, MD (DVD from The Cancer Project's Nutrition & Cancer Video Series)

NEWSLETTERS

Cancer Project News is a quarterly publication distributed by The Cancer Project. To subscribe, go to *www.CancerProject.org* or call 202-244-5038.

E-NEWS

Breaking Medical News is a free service of The Cancer Project and the Physicians Committee for Responsible Medicine, bringing you news from the latest research studies, often before they are available through Medline or other computerized retrieval systems.

Cancer Project News is distributed electronically each quarter.

Recipe of the Week is a weekly e-mail that provides one delicious, healthful recipe per week.

To subscribe to any of the above e-news services, go to *www.CancerProject.org* or call 202-244-5038.

WEB SITES

www.CancerProject.org

Discover The Cancer Project's nationwide Food For Life Nutrition & Cooking Classes for Cancer Prevention and Survival, the latest cancer and nutrition research, Nutrition & Cancer webcasts, and educational resources.

www.NutritionMD.org

Helps health care providers and individuals adopt health-promoting diets by providing nutrition information, research, hundreds of recipe suggestions, and answers for health-related questions.

www.PCRM.org

Learn about diet as preventative medicine for numerous other health conditions and diseases through the vast resources of the Physicians Committee for Responsible Medicine.

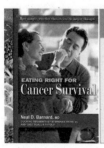

Eating Right for Cancer Survival 2-disk DVD set

This groundbreaking new DVD set is designed to work hand-in-hand with the companion *The Cancer Survivor's Guide.* Together they'll provide you with empowering information on how simple, everyday choices can cause major changes in your health and well being. Contains nine presentations by Neal Barnard, MD, and nine cooking segments by Stephanie Beine, RD, and Chef Sualua Tupolo.

103 mins. • *$19.95*   Order at **www.pcrm.org/shop/** or 800-695-2241

INDEX

A

a-carotene, *55*
acorn squash, *36*
acrylamide, 69
additives, 66, 80
adolescents' diet, 71–72
adrenal glands, 43, 48
African diet, 1
aging process, 30
alcohol, 25, 69
allicin, 35
allium vegetables, 34, 35, *35.*
    See also specific types of
almond milk
    as alternative/substitute, 23,
        63, 67
    calcium in, 20, 22, 58, 72
    shakes from, for weight con-
        trol, 83
    shopping for, 66
almonds
    antioxidants in, *38*
    calcium in, *21,* 58
    Collard Greens with, 176
    as ingredient, in main dish
        recipe, 188
*Aloo Gobi (Potato and Cauli-
    flower Curry),* 197
alpha-linoleic/-linolenic acid,
    75, 88
aluminum cookware,
    Alzheimer's disease and,
    73
Ambrosia, 213
American diet. *See* Western
    (North American) diet
American Dietetic Association,
    26
American Institute for Cancer
    Research, 70
*American Journal of Clinical
    Nutrition, 21,* 70
amino acids
    as building block, 86
    carbohydrates from, 85
    protein and, 22, 86
    in vegan diet, 79, *85,* 87
animal fats/products/protein
    amount consumed, 79
    avoiding, 42, 44, 45
    calcium and, 22, 45, 71, 72
    in children's diet, 71

cholesterol in, 40
    fiber in, lack of, 10
    immune system affected by,
        40
    prostate cancer and, 54
anthocyanins, 32
antibodies, 38
antioxidants
    about, 29–30
    anthocyanins, 32
    in beans and legumes, 37
    beta-carotene, 30
    as cancer fighters, ix, 29
    in children's diet, 71
    cooking's effect on, 73
    in fruits, 37
    in green tea, 83
    immune system and, 38–39
    lycopene, 31
    meal planning for, 41–42
    minimum daily target, 35
    in nuts/oils/seeds, 38
    in plant foods, ix, 30, 79
    prostate cancer and, 55
    selenium, 32
    in vegetables, 29, *29, 36,* 40
    vitamin C, 33
    vitamin E, 32
    in whole grains, *36*
Any Veggie Coconut Curry, 187
appetizers
    Caviar, Texas, 117
    Chips, Baked Tortilla, 106
    Dip, Black Bean, 107
    Dip, Creamy Spinach, 109
    Guacamole, Low-Fat, 110
    *Hummus, Roasted Red Pep-
        per,* 113
    Mushrooms, Stuffed, 116
    *Potato Boats with Spinach
        Stuffing,* 112
    Salsa, Colorful Corn, 108
    Salsa, Mango, 111
    Soybean Snacks (Edamame),
        115
    *Spread with Sun-Dried
        Tomatoes, White Bean,*
        119
    *Sweet Potato Wedges,
        Roasted,* 114
    Veggies in a Blanket, 118
apple(s)

antioxidants in, *37*
    fat in, *4*
    fiber and, 46
    as ingredient, in dessert
        recipe, 216
    juice, as ingredient, in
        recipes, 200, 222
    in New Four Food Groups,
        59
    pesticides in, *64*
    -sauce
        as alternative/substitute,
            67, 74
        Berry, 214
        fiber and, 11
        in hot cereals, 60
        Muffins 1, 96
    as snack, 82
    in study, 50
apricots
    antioxidants in, *37*
    as ingredient, in breakfast
        recipe, 94
    as ingredient, in dessert
        recipe, 221
Argentinian study, 75
arrhythmia, 70
artichoke(s)
    in New Four Food Groups,
        59
    Stew, Lentil, 126
Asia/Asian
    diet, 5, 80
    Fusion Salad, 135
    groceries, 41
    Persuasion Coleslaw, 172
asparagus, *64*
atherosclerosis, 75
Australian study, 49–50
avocados
    avoiding/limiting, 5, 46
    for children/adolescents, 71
    Guacamole, 110
    pesticides in, *64*

B

bacteria
    fiber metabolized by, 86
    food safety and, 76
    lactose and, 19
    vitamin B$_{12}$ and, 59
    white blood cells and, 38

Baked Tofu, 186
Baked Tortilla Chips, 106
bakery items, 66
Balsamic Vinaigrette, 152
banana(s)
    antioxidants in, *37*
    -Date Muffins, 97
    freezing, 100
    as ingredient, in breakfast
        recipe, 95
    as ingredient, in dessert
        recipe, 213
    as ingredient, in smoothie
        recipes
        Blueberry, 100
        Green Goodie, 101
        Green Tea, 103
        Mixed Berry, 102
        Orange Julius, 103
        Strawberry, 104
        Tropical Freeze, 102
    in New Four Food Groups,
        59
    -Oat Pancakes, 91
    pesticides in, *64*
    as snack, 82
    as substitute for oil, 74
barley
    antioxidants in, *36*
    Brown Rice and, 161
    cooking, *15*
    fiber in, 10
    in healthy meal planning,
        60, 61
    in New Four Food Groups,
        59
    selenium in, *33, 41*
    Soup, Mushroom, 129
    vitamin E in, *33, 41*
Barnard, N. D., *21*
Basic Polenta, 160
Basic White Sauce, 157
Basil Salad, Citrus, 138
*Basil Salad, Tomato, Cucum-
    ber, and,* 150
basmati rice
    Brown Rice, 159
    cooking, *15*
    as ingredient, in dessert
        recipe, 221
    Pilaf, Brown Rice, 165
    Pilaf, Rice and Carrot, 169

Pudding, Rice, 221
b-carotene, 55
bean(s) (legumes). See also specific types of
alpha-linoleic acid in, 75
amino acids in, 79
amount recommended, 5, 5, 59, 63
antioxidants in, 37
beta-carotene in, 37
Burritos, Quick, 207
calcium in
amount of, 21
as healthful source, 20, 22, 58, 71
for children/adolescents, 72
calories in, 44
canned, 13, 14
in children's diet, 71
Chili, Three Bean, 132
complex carbohydrates in, 85
cooking, 13
dietary fat vs., 4, 4
dried, 13, 13, 14
fat in, 44, 81
fiber in, 46, 82, 86
grains as accompaniment to, 16
in high-fiber diet, 10, 13
as ingredient, in appetizer recipes, 117, 118
as ingredient, in dip recipe, 109
as ingredient, in hummus recipe, 113
as ingredient, in main dish recipe, 194
as ingredient, in salad recipes, 137, 141, 142
as ingredient, in soup recipe, 122
as ingredient, in stew recipes, 125, 131
iron in, 72
in low-carbohydrate, high-protein diets, 44
as low-fat food, 26
macrobiotic diet and, 78
in meal planning, 61
in New Four Food Groups, 5, 5, 59
omega-3 fatty acids in, 88
prostate cancer and, 57
prostate cancer study and, 55
protein in
amino acids and, 79, 87

amount of, 58, 87, 88
as healthful source, 26–27
Quick Fiber Check and, 11
refried, 27
as replacement, 27, 67
Salad, Easy, 140
Salad, Southwest, 147
sample meal ideas, 60–62
selenium in, 33, 33, 37, 41
serving sizes, 59, 63
shopping for, 14–15, 66
soaking, 14
sodium and, 13, 14
supplements vs., 82
vitamin C in, 37
vitamin E in, 33, 37, 41
bean sprouts
as ingredient, in appetizer recipe, 118
as ingredient, in grain side dish recipe, 167
as ingredient, in salad recipe, 135
beef. See under meat
Beet Salad, Hot or Cold, 143
bell peppers. See also specific types of
as healthful ingredient, 62
as ingredient, in side dish recipe, 182
as ingredient, in taco recipe, 210
pesticides in, 64
in salads, 82
vitamins in, 82
berry(ies). See also specific types of
Applesauce, 214
-Banana Smoothie, Mixed, 102
as ingredient, in salad recipe, 148
as ingredient, in smoothie recipe, 103
shopping for, 66
beta-carotene
about, 30–31, 31
amount of, caution about, 77
breast cancer and, 50
cooking's effect on, 73
as free radical fighter, 30
immune system and, ix, 30, 39
meal planning and, 42
minimum daily target, 35
in plant foods, 36, 37, 38, 41
beverages. See specific types of

black bean(s)
antioxidants in, 37
Brown Rice and, 166
Chili, 121
Chili, Three Bean, 132
cooking, 13
digesting, 14
Dip, 107
as ingredient, in salad recipes, 137, 141
as ingredient, in side dish recipe, 182
as ingredient, in taco recipe, 208
in New Four Food Groups, 59
protein in, 87
and Tomatoes, Spicy, 181
black currant oil, 75
black-eyed peas
antioxidants in, 37
cooking, 13
digesting, 14
as ingredient, in appetizer recipe, 117
as ingredient, in salad recipes, 140, 142
shopping for, 66
bladder cancer, 69, 75–76
Blanket, Veggies in a, 118
blood pressure, 44
blueberry(ies)
anthocyanins in, 32
antioxidants in, 37
as ingredient, in dessert recipe, 214
in New Four Food Groups, 59
nutrients in, 63
Smoothie, 100
vitamin E in, 41
BMI (body mass index), 47
Boats with Spinach Stuffing, Potato, 112
body mass index (BMI), 47
borage oil, 75
Braised Kale, 173
Brazil nuts
antioxidants in, 38
as ingredient, in salad recipe, 148
selenium in, 33
in vegetable salad, 41
vitamin E in, 33
breakfast/breakfast recipes
French Toast, Tofu, 95
in healthy meal planning, 46, 65
Home Fries, Breakfast, 92

Muffins 1, Applesauce, 96
Muffins, Banana-Date, 97
Muffins, Sweet Potato, 98
Pancakes, Banana-Oat, 91
protein and, 87
Quinoa, Fruited Breakfast, 94
sample menu ideas, 59–60
Scramble, 93
breast cancer
alcohol increasing risk of, 69, 69
caffeine consumption and, 70
children's nutrition and, 72
cholesterol's effect on, 51
combined diet and, 50–52
cruciferous vegetables and, 34–35
dairy consumption's role in, viii, 18, 19–20
dietary fats' role in, 3, 48–49
estrogens and, 2
exercise and, 51, 52, 84
fiber's effect on, 49, 51
foods' role in survival of, 47–52, 84
fruit consumption and, 49–50, 51
in Japanese women vs. Western women, 47, 47
menarche and, 72
plant-based diet's effect on, 72
soy consumption and, 27, 80, 81
studies, 43, 47–52
vegetable consumption and, 49–50, 51
vitamin E and, 32
weight's effect on
fatty foods and, 40
healthy foods and, 83–84
studies about, 43, 47–48, 51
breastfeeding, 79
broccoli
à la King, 188
antioxidants in, 36
calcium in, 21
as cancer fighter, 34, 35, 77
cooking, 11, 35
as cruciferous vegetable, 34, 34
digesting, 35
fat in, 4
as ingredient, in main dish recipe, 187
as ingredient, in side dish recipe, 182

as ingredient, in soup recipe, 128

in meal planning, 41, 42, 61

in New Four Food Groups, 59

or Cauliflower with Sesame Salt, 174

pesticides in, 64

phytochemicals in, 34

Salad, 136

in salads, 82

Sauté, Tempeh, 201

shopping for, 66

Soup, Cream of, 122

sulforaphane in, 34

vitamins in, 34, 82

Brown Gravy, Simple, 157

brown rice

antioxidants in, 36

and Barley, 161

with Black Beans, 166

and Carrot Pilaf, 169

cooking, 15

fat in, 4

fiber in, 16

as ingredient, in grain side dish recipe, 169

as ingredient, in main dish recipes, 199, 204

as ingredient, in salad recipe, 142

in New Four Food Groups, 59

Pilaf, 165

recipe for, 159

selenium in, 33

shopping for, 66

Soup, Lentil and, 127

toasting, 163

vitamin E in, 33

brussels sprouts

antioxidants in, 36

as cruciferous vegetable, 34

in meal planning, 42

selenium in, 33

vitamin E in, 33

Buckwheat Pasta with Seitan, 189

bulgur

Fried, Chinese, 167

as ingredient, in appetizer recipe, 117

as ingredient, in main dish recipes, 195, 204

in New Four Food Groups, 59

and Orange Salad, 137

Pilaf, Tex-Mex, 170

recipe for, 162

Salad, Lentil and, 144

burgers. See sandwiches/burgers/wraps

Burritos, Quick Bean, 207

butternut squash, as ingredient, in side dish recipe, 182

butter substitutes, 67

C

cabbage

antioxidants in, 36

calcium in, 21

as cancer fighter, 41, 77

Coleslaw, Asian Persuasion, 172

cooking, for digestion, 11

as cruciferous vegetable, 34, 34

in meal planning, 61

phytochemicals in, 34

red, anthocyanin in, 32

caffeine, 69–70, 71

Calabacitas, 175

calcium

absorption rate, 21, 70

amount recommended, 21, 70–71

breast cancer and, 19–20

caffeine consumption affecting, 70

cancer and, 18–20

in children's diet, 72

colon cancer and, 19

in cow's milk, 18, 19, 70

in cow's milk alternatives, 20

in dairy products, viii, 19

in greens, 58

loss, 80

in plant foods, 20, 21, 21, 70

prostate cancer and, 19–20

sources of, 20–22, 21, 70, 71

supplements, 20

in urine, 45

vitamin D and, 18, 19, 20

calories

carbohydrates and, 86

in Daily Diet, 63

dietary fat and

amount of, 7, 74, 88

in foods

beef, 3

eggs, 75

lack of, in healthful foods, 44

list of, 4

soy products, 81

studies about, 2–3, 51

exercise to burn, 45

low-fat diets and, 49

plant foods and, 44, 46, 83

protein and, 58, 79, 87, 87

in soy products, 81

in sugars, 82

Canadian study, 50

Cancer Prevention Study II, 25

Cancer Project, The, 89

canned goods

beans, 13, 14, 14–15

in healthy meal planning, 42, 46, 62, 66

sodium and, 13, 22

canola oil, 54, 88

cantaloupe

antioxidants in, 30, 37

beta-carotene in, 31

Gingered Melon, 218

in healthy meal planning, 6, 46, 60

vitamin C in, 34

carbohydrates, 85–86, 88

carbon dioxide, 29

carcinogens

allium/cruciferous vegetables to remove, 34, 35

fiber to remove, 10

heterocyclic amines (HCAs), 10, 78

in pesticides/fertilizers, 64

polycyclic aromatic hydrocarbons, 69

cardiac arrhythmia, 70

carotenoids, 31, 41, 51, 55

carrot(s)

antioxidants in, 36

beta-carotene in, 31, 41, 73

cooking's effect on, 73

as ingredient, in appetizer recipe, 118

as ingredient, in main dish recipes, 187, 200

as ingredient, in salad recipes, 135, 136

as ingredient, in side dish recipes, 172, 182

as ingredient, in soup recipe, 123

as ingredient, in stew recipes, 125, 131

Pilaf, Rice and, 169

in salads, 82

vitamins in, 82

cashews

antioxidants in, 38

as ingredient, in appetizer recipes, 112, 116

as ingredient, in main dish recipes, 188, 194

as ingredient, in sauce recipe, 157

Casserole, Red Bean, 199

cast iron cookware, 73

catechins, 83

cauliflower

antioxidants in, 36

calcium in, 21

cooking, for digestion, 11

as cruciferous vegetable, 34

Curry (Aloo Gobi), Potato and, 197

in healthy meal planning, 41, 61

Mashed Grains and, 168

in New Four Food Groups, 59

pesticides in, 64

with Sesame Salt, Broccoli or, 174

Caviar, Texas, 117

celery

as ingredient, in burger recipe, 204

as ingredient, in main dish recipes, 195, 198, 199, 200

as ingredient, in salad recipes, 142, 145, 147

as ingredient, in sauce recipe, 155

as ingredient, in side dish recipes, 167, 172

as ingredient, in soup recipe, 133

as ingredient, in stew recipes, 125, 131

as ingredient, in wrap recipe, 205

pesticides in, 64

as snack, 62

cereal. See also oatmeal/oat(s)

Bulgur, 162

calcium and, 22

fiber and, 6, 10, 11, 46

flaxseeds added to, 75

in New Four Food Groups, 59

nondairy alternatives for, 20, 22, 23, 59

protein in, 87

sample breakfast ideas, 59–60

sample snack idea, 62

serving sizes, 63

vitamin B_{12} in, 59, 71, 82

zinc in, 39

cheese (dairy)

alternatives for, 22, 23, 46,
64
avoiding/eliminating, 62, 76
cancer risk and, 19
cost of, vs. vegetarian
choice, 73–74
fat in, viii
cherries
anthocyanins in, 32
as ingredient, in smoothie
recipe, 101
pesticides in, 64
chicken. See under poultry
chickpea(s)
antioxidants in, 37
Burgers, 204
cooking, 13
fiber in, for healthy weight,
46
Hummus, Roasted Red Pep-
per, 113
as ingredient, in main dish
recipe, 187
as ingredient, in side dish
recipe, 182
as ingredient, in stew recipe,
131
in New Four Food Groups,
59
protein in, 87
Salad Romaine Wraps, 205
selenium in, 33
shopping for, 66
vitamin E in, 33
zinc in, 39
children's diet, 71–72
chili beans, as ingredient, in
salad recipe, 147
chili/chiles
Black Bean, 121
as ingredient, in appetizer
recipes, 111, 117
as ingredient, in main dish
recipe, 192
as ingredient, in side dish
recipes, 181, 184
as ingredient, in soup recipe,
130
as ingredient, in stew recipe,
131
as ingredient, in taco recipe,
210
as ingredient, in wrap recipe,
209
Three Bean, 132
Chinese food/medicine/studies,
47, 68, 78, 83
Fried Bulgur, 167
Chips, Baked Tortilla, 106

chocolate
almond/rice milks, 23
Mousse or Chocolate
Mousse Pie, 215
saturated fat in, 48
cholesterol
in animal products, 42, 79
breast cancer affected by, 51
in dairy products, viii
fiber's effect on, 86
guidelines for, 7
immune system and, ix, 40
lack of, in vegetarian diet, 40
soluble fiber and, 10
soy consumption affecting,
81
chromosomes, 30, 86
Chunky Ratatouille Sauce, 155
citrus fruit
Basil Salad, 138
in New Four Food Groups,
59
nutrients in, 63
Spinach Salad with, 148
coconut
avoiding/limiting, 46
Curry, Any Veggie, 187
fat in, 46, 74, 88
as ingredient, in dessert
recipes, 213, 221
coconut oil, 88
coffee, 58, 69–70
Cold Beet Salad, Hot or, 143
Coleslaw, Asian Persuasion,
172
colitis, 75, 88
collagen, 21
collard greens
with Almonds, 176
calcium in, 21
as cancer fighter, 41
as cruciferous vegetable, 34
in meal planning, 42
in New Four Food Groups,
59
phytochemicals in, 34
Zippy Yams and, 184
colon cancer
allium vegetables' effect on,
35
calcium to reduce risk of, 19
coffee consumption decreasing risk of, 69
fiber to reduce risk of, 10
meat consumption's role in,
25, 26, 45
study, 25–26
whole grains to protect
against, 38

colorectal cancer, 25, 69, 75, 83
Colorful Corn Salsa, 108
combining foods, 27, 79, 87
Community Supported Agriculture (CSA), 78
complex carbohydrates, 77,
85–86
Compote, Summer Fruit, 222
condiments, 6, 58
constipation, 10, 11, 13
cooking food, 72–73, 79–80
cookware, 73
corn
as ingredient, in grain side
dish recipe, 170
as ingredient, in main dish
recipe, 192
as ingredient, in salad
recipes, 140, 141, 147
as ingredient, in side dish
recipe, 175
in meal planning, 61
pesticides in, 64
Salsa, Colorful, 108
shopping for, 66
corn grits recipe (Basic Polenta),
160
cornmeal
cooking, 15
as ingredient, in dessert
recipe, 219
corn oil, 75
cost of healthful eating, 73, 74
cottonseed oil, 75
couscous
cooking, 15
Grains and Cauliflower,
Mashed, 168
in healthy meal planning,
60, 61
as ingredient, in main dish
recipes, 190, 192, 201
in New Four Food Groups,
59
recipe for, 163
toasting, 163
cranberries, as ingredient, in
dessert recipe, 216
cranberry juice, as ingredient,
in smoothie recipe, 103
cream cheese, substitutes for, 67
cream substitutes, 67
creamy dishes
Dip, Spinach, 109
Dressing, Dill, 153
Soup, Cream of Broccoli, 122
Soup, Root, 123
cruciferous vegetables. See also
specific types of

cancer-fighting effect of,
34–35, 77
cooking, 11
in healthy meal planning,
41, 42
list of, 34
CSA (Community Supported
Agriculture), 78
cucumber
and Basil Salad, Tomato,
150
in healthy meal planning,
46, 60
as ingredient, in salad
recipes, 135, 138, 144
in New Four Food Groups,
59
Salad, Mango and Spinach,
139
Curry, Any Veggie Coconut,
187
Curry (Aloo Gobi), Potato and
Cauliflower, 197
Custard, Pumpkin Pie or, 220
cyanocobalamin, 59, 72

D
Daily Diet Checklist, 63
dairy products. See also specific
types of
alternatives to, viii, 17–23, 64
in Asian diet, 81
avoiding, 5, 58, 68, 76–77
bacteria in, 76
calcium in, viii, 70
calories in, 44
cancer and, viii, 1, 17
cholesterol in, 78
fat in, 48, 52, 54, 78
fiber in, lack of, 10
IGF-1 and, 78
nutrients in, lack of, 70
prostate cancer and, 53, 57
Quick Fiber Check and, 11
Date Muffins, Banana-, 97
desserts
Ambrosia, 213
Applesauce, Berry, 214
Fruit Compote, Summer,
222
Gingerbread, 217
Melon, Gingered, 218
Mousse, Chocolate, or
Chocolate Mousse Pie,
215
Pie or Custard, Pumpkin,
220
Pudding, Harvest, 219
Pudding, Rice, 221

Pudding, Tapioca, 223
sample ideas, 62
Yams, Festive Fruited, 216
diabetes
  in children, 71
  diet's effect on, x, 44
  fiber and, 13, 86
  weight and, 44
diet(s). *See also* specific types
    of
  for adolescents/children,
      71–72
  calcium in, 58
  Daily Diet Checklist, 63
  Dietary Reference Intakes, 36
  Diet Record form, 6, 8
  dining out and, 68
  getting started/meal planning,
      64–65, 65
  grocery shopping for, 65, 66
  organic foods for, 64
  protein in, 58
  record for, 6–7
  risky, 44–45
  role in cancer, ix–x, 1–3
  sample meals, 59–62
  significant vs. insignificant
      changes in, 2–3
  substitutions, 67, 67
  three-week break, 57, 57–58,
      77
  vitamin B$_{12}$ in, 59
digestive problems
  with beans, 14
  constipation, 10, 11, 13
  with cruciferous vegetables,
      11, 35
  fiber and, 9, 11, 13
Dill Dressing, Creamy, 153
dining out, 68
dinner
  in healthy meal planning, 6,
      46, 64, 65
  protein and, 87
  sample menu ideas, 61–62
  in 3-3-3 revamping of diet, x
Dip, Black Bean, 107
Dip, Creamy Spinach, 109
DNA, 26, 30
dried apricots, as ingredient, in
    dessert recipe, 221
dried beans
  cooking/soaking, 13, 13, 14
  in healthy meal planning,
      14–15
  shopping for, 66
  for weight gain, 83
dried coconut, as ingredient, in
    dessert recipe, 221

dried cranberries, as ingredient,
    in recipes, 136, 213, 216
dried fruits
  Australian study, 50
  as snack, 62, 65, 82
  for weight control, 83
dried peas, for weight gain, 83
dry goods, 66

E

Easy Bean Salad, 140
Easy Stir-Fry, 190
eating out, 68
Edamame (Soybean Snacks),
    115
egg(s)
  avoiding, 5, 58
  bacteria in, 76
  bladder cancer and, 75–76
  calories in, 44
  cholesterol in, 75
  colorectal cancer and, 75
  fiber in, lack of, 10, 75
  prostate cancer and, 57
  Quick Fiber Check and, 11
  saturated fat in, 48, 75
  studies, 75
  substitutes for, 67, 76
  tofu as substitute for, in
      breakfast recipes, 93, 95
  whites, 75, 76, 77
eggplant
  in healthy meal planning,
      60, 62, 67
  as ingredient, in sauce recipe,
      155
  as ingredient, in side dish
      recipe, 182
  Lasagne, 191
  Ratatouille Sauce, Chunky,
      155
electrons, 29
English meat studies, 25
enterohepatic circulation, 9
entrées. *See* main dishes
Environmental Working
    Group, 64, 64
essential amino acids, 86
essential fatty acids, 74–75, 88
estradiol, 2, 35
estrogen
  about, 1–2
  cancer cell growth and, 48
  cookware and, 73
  cruciferous vegetables and,
      34–35
  diet's effect on, viii, 1
  fiber's effect on, 49
  low-fat diet and, 49, 53

prostate cancer and, 55
soy and, 80, 81
weight and, 43, 43
European diet, 17, 81
evening primrose oil, 75
exercise
  for bone health, 20
  breast cancer and, 51, 52
  cancer and, 4
  healthy weight and, 45, 46
  New Four Food Groups'
      diet vs., 44
  prostate cancer and, 54, 55
  protein requirements and, 87
  recommendation about, 70
  studies, 52, 55

F

fad diets, 44–45
fast food restaurants, 68
fat (body), 43, 43, 48. *See also*
    obesity; weight
fat (dietary)
  amount recommended, 88
  avoiding/limiting, 74
  breast cancer and, 48–49
  calories in, 44, 49, 88
  cancer and, 1, 2
  in children's diet, 71
  cholesterol vs., 40
  in dairy products, viii
  death increased by, 3
  estrogen affected by, 51
  guidelines for, 7
  immune system and, ix
  lowering, for health, 88
  monounsaturated, 54, 88
  necessity of, 88
  omega-3/omega-6 fatty
      acids, 74–75
  polyunsaturated, 88
  protein in, lack of, 87
  recommendation, 89
  saturated
    about, 88
    in chicken/fish, 76
    in children's diet, 71
    in eggs, 75
    in North American diet, 79
    in organic dairy products/
        meat, 78
    in plant-derived omega-
        3s, 75
    in plant foods, 74
    studies about, 48, 54
  in specific foods
    animal products, 42, 79,
        88
    beef, 3

chicken, 3, 26, 88
meat, viii, 26, 88
milk, 17, 18
plant foods vs. other
    foods, 3–5, 4
soybeans, 81
studies, 2–3, 4
substitutes for, 64–65
types of, 88
fatty acids, 74–75, 81, 88
fatty foods/diets
  avoiding/eliminating, 5, 58
  breast cancer and, 48
  immune system affected by,
      40
  prostate cancer and, 53
Festive Fruited Yams, 216
*Fettuccine, Mushroom
    Stroganoff over,* 194
fiber
  amount recommended,
      10–11, 49, 86
  benefits of, 77, 86
  calorie intake affected by, 44
  cancer and, 49, 53
  in children's diet, 71
  estrogen affected by, 51
  healthy weight and, 45–46
  insoluble, 10–11, 86
  lack of, in foods, 9, 10, 18
  in plant foods, 44, 81, 82,
      86
  as preventive
    for cancer, viii, 11, 26
    for health problems, 13
    for hormone circulation, 9
  role of, 9
  soluble, 10, 81, 86
  in soy/soy products, 81
fibrocystic breast disease, 70
Fiesta Salad, 141
figs
  in children's diet, 72
  non-plant foods vs., 58
  prostate cancer and, 71
  serving size for, 21
  as snack, 22
fish
  cholesterol in, 76
  essential fatty acids and,
      74–75
  fat in, 3–4, 4, 76, 88
  fiber in, lack of, 10
  heterocyclic amines (HCAs)
      and, 78
  omega-3 fatty acids in, 75
  Quick Fiber Check and, 11
  substitutes for, 67
fish oil, 75

flaxseed oil, 75
flaxseeds, *38*, 75, 88
folic acid, 69
food additives, 66, 80
food combining, 27, 79, 87
food safety, 76
foods' role in fighting cancer, vii–x
free radicals, 29–30, 69
Freeze, Tropical, 102
French Toast, Tofu, 95
Fried Bulgur, Chinese, 167
fried foods
    avoiding, 5, 58
    cancer risk and, 2, 3, 56
    estrogen increased by, 1
    plant foods vs., 44
Fries, Breakfast Home, 92
frozen foods, 66
fruit(s). *See also* specific types of
    alpha-linoleic acid in, 75
    Ambrosia, 213
    amount recommended
        in Daily Diet Checklist, *63*
        in New Four Food Groups, 5, *5*, 59
        whole vs. juiced, 77
    antioxidants in, 29, *29*
    calcium and, 72
    calories in, 44
    cancer and, 49–50, 53, 55, 57
    as canned good, 66
    in children's diet, 71
    Compote, Summer, 222
    cooking's effect on, 79–80
    dietary fat vs., 4, *4*
    fat in, 44
    fiber and, 10, 46, 82, 86
    frozen, 66
    as low-fat food, 26
    in meal planning, 41
    in New Four Food Groups, 5, *5*
    omega-3 fatty acids in, 88
    pesticides in, 64
    phytochemicals in, 29, *29*
    and Pine Nuts, Salad of Spicy Greens with, 146
    Quick Fiber Check and, 11
    Quinoa, Fruited Breakfast, 94
    sample meal ideas, 59–62
    serving sizes, 59, *63*
    shopping for, 66
    as snack, 82
    supplements vs., 82
    vitamin C in, 21, 33, 72
    washing, 76
    Yams, Festive Fruited, 216

Fusion Salad, Asian, 135

G
galactose, 19
gamma-linolenic acid, 75
garlic
    antioxidants in, *36*
    as cancer fighter, 35, 36
    cooking's effect on, 35
    Mashed Potatoes, 177
    in meal planning, 42
    roasted, *160*
    selenium in, *33*
    studies, 35
    vitamin E in, *33*
gastric cancer, 83
genistein, 81
German Cancer Research Center, 40
German study, 25
ginger(ed)
    -bread, 217
    as ingredient, in dessert recipes, 219, 220
    as ingredient, in main dish recipes, 186, 201
    as ingredient, in side dish recipes, 167, 169, 172
    as ingredient, in soup recipe, 128
    as ingredient, in stew recipe, 131
    Melon, 218
glucose, 19, 85
glycogen, 85
grains. *See* whole grains
grapefruit
    antioxidants in, 37
    as ingredient, in salad recipe, 148
    lycopene in
        amount of, *32*, 37
        as cancer fighter, 55
        choosing, at grocery store, 42
        as pigment, 31
grapes
    antioxidants in, 37
    in Australian study, 50
    as ingredient, in salad recipe, 148
    in New Four Food Groups, 59
    pesticides in, 64
Gravy, Mushroom, 156
Gravy, Simple Brown, 157
great northern beans
    calcium in, *21*
    cooking, *13*

as ingredient, in chili recipe, 132
green beans
    in ethnic meals, 68
    as ingredient, in stew recipe, 125
    in New Four Food Groups, 59
green bell pepper
    as ingredient, in appetizer recipes, 108, 117
    as ingredient, in breakfast recipe, 92
    as ingredient, in chili recipes, 121, 132
    as ingredient, in grain side dish recipe, 166
    as ingredient, in main dish recipes, 195, 200
    as ingredient, in salad recipes, 141, 147
    as ingredient, in stew recipe, 125
Green Goodie Smoothie, 101
greens. *See also* specific types of
    beta-carotene in, 30
    calcium in
        absorption rate, *70*
        amount of, *21,* 71
        for children, 72
        in healthy meal planning, 22, 58
    as cancer fighter, 41
    cooking, 42
    as cruciferous vegetables, *34*
    dinner ideas for, 61
    with Fruit and Pine Nuts, Salad of Spicy, 146
    iron in, 72
green tea, 83
    Smoothie, 103
Grilled Plantains, 177
grilling meat/chicken, 26, 78
grocery shopping, 65, 66
Guacamole, Low-Fat, 110
guar gum, 86
guava, *34, 37, 55*

H
Harvard Nurses' Health Study, 19
Harvard University, viii, 17, 19, 20, 31, 72
HCAs (heterocyclic amines), viii, 10, 26, 78
Health Professionals Follow-Up Study, viii
Heaney, R., *21*
heart disease

alcohol and, 69
    Asian diet and, 81
    in children, 71
    dietary fats' effect on, 88
    diet's effect on, 44, 54
    essential fatty acids and, 88
    fiber as preventive for, 13, 86
    Japanese diet and, 71
    omega fatty acids to protect against, 75
Heinz Institute of Nutritional Sciences, 32
hempseed oil, 75
heterocyclic amines (HCAs), viii, 10, 26, 78
high-fat diet/foods
    avoiding, 5, 58
    cancer/hormones affected by, 1, 45
    dairy products, 2
    meat, viii, 2
    plants foods vs., 73
high-fiber diet/foods
    amount of, 10
    cancer affected by, viii, 10, 26, 53
    cooking, 13
    estrogen affected by, 2
    meat, 26
    in study, 51
    vegetarians and, 86
    for weight loss, 45–46
high-protein diets, 44–45
Home Fries, Breakfast, 92
Home-Style Squash and Pinto Beans, 192
Hong Kong study, 53, *53*
Hoppin' John Salad, 142
hormones
    cancer and
        foods influencing, viii, 1, *1*
        weight affecting, 43, *43,* 48
    cruciferous vegetables and, 34–35
    in dairy products/milk, 17, 78
    dietary fat and, 51, 88
    diet as booster to, 26
    fiber and, 9, 51
    insulin-like growth factor (IGF-1), 18, 19, 53, 78
Hot or Cold Beet Salad, 143
hummus
    fiber in, for healthy weight, 46
    in healthy meal planning, 6, 41, 60

as ingredient, in appetizer recipe, 118
Roasted Red Pepper, 113
shopping for, 66
as snack, 62, 65
hypertension, x, 80

I

ice cream, 22, 23, 76
IGF-1 (insulin-like growth factor)
  as breast cancer risk, viii, 18, 19
  in dairy products, viii, 18, *18,* 78
  as prostate cancer risk, viii, 18, 53
immune system
  antioxidants as aid to, 38–39
  body fat's effect on, 43
  cholesterol and, ix, 40
  fatty foods effect on, 40
  fiber assisting, viii
  healthy meal planning and, 41–42
  role in fighting cancer, ix
  vegetarian diet and, 40–41
  zinc and, 39, *39*
Indian food, 68
Indian Seasoning Mix, 183
indole-3-carbinol, 35
Institute of Medicine, 30
insulin, 82
insulin-like growth factor (IGF-1). *See* IGF-1 (insulin-like growth factor)
international foods, 68
International Urology and Nephrology, 76
iodine, 80
iron, in children's diet, 72
isoflavones, 81
isothiocyanates, 77
Italian food, 68
Italian Seasoning Mix, 183

J

Japanese diet/food
  breast cancer and, 47, *47*
  children's, 71
  in healthy diet, 68
  Western influence on, 1
jasmine rice
  Brown Rice, 159
  Pilaf, Brown Rice, 165
  Pilaf, Rice and Carrot, 169
  Pudding, Rice, 221
joint pain/problems, 45, 75, 88

Journal of the American Dietetic Association, 21, 70
Journal of the American Medical Association, 52
Journal of the National Cancer Institute, 2
juices/juicing, 58, 71, 72, 77. *See also* specific types of juices
Julius, Orange, 103

K

kale
  antioxidants in, *36*
  beta-carotene in, *31*
  Braised, 173
  calcium in, *21*
  as cancer fighter, 41
  as cruciferous vegetable, *34*
  as ingredient, in main dish recipe, 187
  in meal planning, 42
  in New Four Food Groups, *59*
  and Potato Soup, Portuguese, 130
  Tomatoes, and Olives, Penne with, 196
Keller, J. L., *21*
kidney beans
  antioxidants in, *37*
  in healthy diet, x, 60
  as ingredient, in salad recipe, 140
  in New Four Food Groups, *59*
  protein in, 87
  shopping for, 66
kiwi, *34, 37, 59, 64*
kombu, 14

L

lactose, 17, 19
Lancet, 77
Lanou, A. J., *21*
Lasagne, Eggplant, 191
Lasagne, Lazy, 193
Latin Seitan Stew, 125
Lazy Lasagne, 193
leeks, *35, 36*
legumes. *See* bean(s) (legumes)
lentil(s)
  antioxidants in, *37*
  Artichoke Stew, 126
  and Brown Rice Soup, 127
  and Bulgur Salad, 144
  calcium in, *20*
  cooking, *13*
  in Daily Diet Checklist, *63*

digesting, 14
fat in, *4*
fiber and, 11
healthy weight and, 46
as meat replacement, 27, 28
in New Four Food Groups, *5, 59,* 60, 72
protein in, *87,* 88
shopping for, 66
soy vs., 81
lettuce
  fiber in, 6
  Romaine Wraps, Chickpea Salad, 205
  in *Salad, Asian Fusion,* 135
lifestyle's role in cancer, vii
lima beans
  cooking, *13*
  in *Salad, Easy Bean,* 140
  shopping for, 15
linoleic/linolenic acids, 74, 75
liver cancer, 69
Loaf, No-Meat, 195
locust bean gum, 86
London study, 26
low-fat diet
  about, 2–3
  breast cancer and, 48–49
  prostate cancer and, 53, 56
  studies, 2–3, 4, 48–49, 54
Low-Fat Guacamole, 110
lunch
  in healthy meal planning, 46, 65
  protein and, 87
  sample menu ideas, 60–61
lung cancer, 77
lutein, 55
lycopene
  about, 31–32
  amount recommended, 56
  cooking's effect on, 73
  in fruits, *32,* 55
  in meal planning, 42
  prostate cancer and, 55
  studies, 55–56
  in tomatoes/tomato products, *32, 36,* 41, 55

M

macrobiotic diet, 54–55, 77–78
macronutrients, 85
main dishes
  Broccoli à la King, 188
  Casserole, Red Bean, 199
  Curry, Any Veggie Coconut, 187
  Curry (Aloo Gobi), Potato and Cauliflower, 197

Lasagne, Eggplant, 191
Lasagne, Lazy, 193
Loaf, No-Meat, 195
Pasta with Seitan, Buckwheat, 189
Penne with Kale, Tomatoes, and Olives, 196
Pilaf, Quinoa, 198
sample dinner ideas, 62
Sauté, Tempeh Broccoli, 201
Squash and Pinto Beans, Home-Style, 192
Stir-Fry, Easy, 190
Stir-Fry, Sweet-and-Sour, 200
Stroganoff over Fettuccine, Mushroom, 194
Tofu, Baked, 186
mango(es)
  antioxidants in, *37*
  beta-carotene in, *31*
  dicing, *111*
  as ingredient, in smoothie recipe, 102
  in New Four Food Groups, *59*
  pesticides in, *64*
  Salsa, 111
  shopping for, 66
  and Spinach Salad, Cucumber, 139
margarine, 5
Marinara Sauce, Simple, 156
mashed foods
  Grains and Cauliflower, 168
  Potatoes, Garlic, 177
  Potatoes, Parsnip, 178
  Potatoes, Rutabaga, 179
mayonnaise, 58, 76
meal planning/sample meals, 41–42, 46, 59–62, 64–65
meat
  alternatives to (*See also* specific types of)
    in Daily Diet Checklist, *63*
    protein needs and, 79
    seitan, 61
    shopping for, 66
    soy-based meats, 64
    suggested, *67*
    vegan sausage/Canadian bacon, 60
    veggie burgers, 64
  in Asian diet, 81
  avoiding/limiting, viii–ix, 5, 58, 76
  bacteria in, 76
  beef
    chicken vs., 3, 4

colon cancer and, 25
fat in, 3, *4*, 40, 88
organic, HCA and, 78
refried beans as substitute
    for, 27
vegetable stew as substi-
    tute for, x
calories in, 44
cancer risk and
    breast cancer, 1
    colon cancer, 25
    increased, viii–ix, 2
    reducing, 26
    in Western diet, 17, *17*
cholesterol in, 78, 79
fat in
    beef, *4*, 88
    saturated, 48, 54, 78, 79
    in study, 52
fiber in, lack of, 10
heterocyclic amines (HCAs)
    and, 78
organic, 78
prostate cancer and, 57
Quick Fiber Check and, 11
replacing, 25–28
studies, 25–26
melon, 59, 60. *See also* specific
    types of
Gingered, 218
menstruation/menstrual pain,
    44, 75, 80, 88
metabolites, 69
Mexican food, 68
Mexican Seasoning Mix, 183
milk (cow's)
    alternatives/substitutes for,
        59, 67
    bacteria in raw, 76
    cancer risk and, 17–20,
        22–23
    fiber in, lack of, 77
    iron in, lack of, 72
    protein in, 27
    whole vs. skim, 22–23, 58
millet
    antioxidants in, *36*
    cooking, 15
    Grains and Cauliflower,
        Mashed, 168
    in healthy meal planning, 61
    as ingredient, in appetizer
        recipes, 112, 116
    as ingredient, in main dish
        recipe, 188
    as ingredient, in sauce recipe,
        157
    as ingredient, in stew recipe,
        125

in New Four Food Groups,
    59
toasting, *163*
minerals, 71, 82
miso soup(s), 68, 80
    with Shiitake Mushrooms,
        128
Mixed Berry Smoothie, 102
monounsaturated fat, 54, 88
Mousse, Chocolate, or Choco-
    late Mousse Pie, 215
Mt. Sinai Medical Center, 51
muffins
    Banana-Date, 97
    1, Applesauce, 96
    Sweet Potato, 98
multivitamins, 39, 42, 46, 72
mushroom(s)
    antioxidants in, *36*
    Barley Soup, 129
    Gravy, 156
    as ingredient, in main dish
        recipes, 188, 189, 191,
        200
    as ingredient, in sauce recipe,
        155
    as ingredient, in side dish
        recipes, 165, 175
    as meat replacement, 27
    portobello, x, 27
        Pan-Seared, 206
    Shiitake, Miso Soup with,
        128
    Stroganoff over Fettuccine,
        194
    Stuffed, 116

N

National Cancer Institute
    (NCI), 48
natural killer (NK) cells, ix,
    40–41
navy beans, *4, 13, 21*, 66
NCI (National Cancer Insti-
    tute), 48
nectarines, pesticides in, *64*
New Four Food Groups
    food examples, 59
    healthy weight with, 44, 45
    meal planning with, 5–6, 58
    servings, *5*, 59
Nicklaus, Jack, vii
NK (natural killer) cells, ix,
    40–41
N-nitroso compounds, 26
No-Meat Loaf, 195
nondairy creamers, 58
nondairy frozen desserts,
    shakes from, 83

nondairy products, 66
nondairy yogurt, viii
North American diet. *See*
    Western (North American)
    diet
nut butters, 5, 71
nutrient analysis/guidelines, 7
Nutrient Data Laboratory, *4,*
    31, 33
nutritional yeast, 22, 59, 72,
    82
nutrition recommendation,
    76–77
nuts. *See also* specific types of
    antioxidants in, *38*
    avoiding/limiting, 5, 46, 58,
        74
    beta-carotene in, *38*
    fat in, 32, 74
    selenium in, *33, 38*, 41
    vitamin C in, *38*
    vitamin E and, 32, *33, 38*
    for weight gain, 83

O

oatmeal/oat(s)
    antioxidants in, *36*
    calcium and, 22
    cooking, 15
    fiber and, 10, 11, 46, 86
    in healthy meal planning, 6,
        60
    as ingredient, in main dish
        recipe, 195
    in New Four Food Groups,
        59
    Pancakes, Banana-, 91
    serving sizes, 59, 63
    shopping for, 66
    weight control and, 46
    when traveling, 65
oat milk
    as alternative/substitute, 20,
        22, 63, 67
    calcium in, 58, 72
    shopping for, 66
obesity, 1, 71
oils, 5, *38*, 40, 49. *See also* spe-
    cific types of
olive oil, *38*, 54
olives
    avoiding/limiting, 5, 46
    Penne with Kale, Tomatoes,
        and, 196
omega-3 fatty acids, 74–75, 81,
    88
omega-6 fatty acids, 74–75, 88
onions, 35, *35, 36*, 64
oral cancer, 83

orange(s)
    antioxidants in, *37*
    fat in, *4*
    as ingredient, in dessert
        recipe, 213
    as ingredient, in salad
        recipes, 138, 148
    as ingredient, in smoothie
        recipes, 102, 103
    Julius, 103
    Radicchio, and Sesame,
        Spinach Salad with, 149
    Salad, Bulgur and, 137
    as snack, 82
    vitamin C in, *34*
orange juice
    antioxidants in, *37*
    calcium in, *21*
    as ingredient, in dessert
        recipes, 213, 216
    as ingredient, in smoothie
        recipe, 103
    vitamin C in, *34*
organic foods, 64, 78–79
Ornish, Dean, 54
osteoporosis, x, 20, 22, 45
ovarian cancer, viii, 19
oxidation, 73
oxygen/oxygen molecules, 29,
    30, 38

P

palm oil, 74, 88
Pancakes, Banana-Oat, 91
pancreatic cancer, 69
Pan-Seared Portobello Mush-
    rooms, 206
papaya, *37, 64*
parsnip(s)
    as ingredient, in side dish
        recipe, 182
    Mashed Potatoes, 178
pasta
    Fettuccine, Mushroom
        Stroganoff over, 194
    as ingredient, in main dish
        recipes, 188, 192
    Lasagne, Lazy, 193
    in low-carbohydrate, high-
        protein diets, 44
    in New Four Food Groups,
        59
    Penne with Kale, Tomatoes,
        and Olives, 196
    protein in, 88
    sauces, 55, 77
    with Seitan, Buckwheat,
        189
    shopping for, 66

Pauling, Linus, 33
peach(es)
    antioxidants in, *37*
    canned, shopping for, *66*
    as ingredient, in dessert
        recipe, 222
    as ingredient, in smoothie
        recipe, 101
    in New Four Food Groups,
        59
    pesticides in, *64*
peanuts
    antioxidants in, *38*
    as ingredient, in side dish
        recipes, 169, 172
pears
    as ingredient, in salad recipe,
        146
    in New Four Food Groups,
        59
    pesticides in, *64*
    as snack, 82
peas
    antioxidants in, *37*
    calcium in, 20
    as ingredient, in appetizer
        recipe, 110
    as ingredient, in grain side
        dish recipe, 170
    as ingredient, in main dish
        recipe, 187
    as ingredient, in stew recipe,
        125
    pesticides in, *64*
    protein in, *87*, 88
    shopping for, *66*
    zinc in, *39*
Pennsylvania State University,
    20
perfluorooctanoic acid (PFOA),
    73
pesticides, 64, *64*, 78, 79
PFOA (perfluorooctanoic acid),
    73
Physicians Committee for
    Responsible Medicine, 5,
    44
Physicians Health Study, viii
phytochemicals
    about, 33–35
    for children, 71
    in foods
        to fight cancer, 29, 76
        grains, 38
        organic, 78
        when meal planning,
            41–42
    in plant foods vs. supple-
        ments, 82

phytoestrogens, 80, 81
*Pie, Chocolate Mousse, or
    Chocolate Mousse,* 215
Pie or Custard, Pumpkin, 220
pilaf
    Brown Rice, 165
    Bulgur, Tex-Mex, 170
    Quinoa, 198
    Rice and Carrot, 169
pineapple(s)
    canned, shopping for, *66*
    as ingredient, in dessert
        recipe, 213
    as ingredient, in grain side
        dish recipe, 169
    as ingredient, in main dish
        recipe, 200
    as ingredient, in stew recipe,
        131
    pesticides in, *64*
*Pine Nuts, Salad of Spicy
    Greens with Fruit and,*
    146
pinto beans
    antioxidants in, *37*
    cooking, *13*
    digesting, 14
    Home-Style Squash and, 192
    as ingredient, in salad recipe,
        140
    as ingredient, in wrap recipe,
        209
    protein in, *87*
    selenium in, *33*
    vitamin E in, *33*
Piquant Dressing, 152
Plantains, Grilled, 177
plant foods
    calcium in, 20, 21, *21*, 70
    cancer prevention and, viii,
        79
    in children's diet, 71
    fiber in, 44, 81, 86
    protein in, 81, *85*, 87
Plawecki, K. L., *21*
Polenta, Basic, 160
polycyclic aromatic hydrocar-
    bons, 69
polyphenolic compounds, 83
polyunsaturated fat, 88
pomegranate juice, as ingredi-
    ent, in smoothie recipe,
    103
porcupine method of dicing,
    111
portobello mushrooms, 27
    Pan-Seared, 206
*Portuguese Kale and Potato
    Soup,* 130

potato(es). *See also* sweet
    potato(es)
    antioxidants in, *36*
    Boats with Spinach Stuffing,
        112
    *and Cauliflower Curry (Aloo
        Gobi),* 197
    complex carbohydrates in,
        85
    Garlic Mashed, 177
    Home Fries, Breakfast, 92
    as ingredient, in main dish
        recipe, 187
    as ingredient, in side dish
        recipe, 182
    as ingredient, in soup recipe,
        123
    as ingredient, in stew recipe,
        125
    Parsnip Mashed, 178
    pesticides in, *64*
    Rutabaga Mashed, 179
    Salad, 145
    Soup, Portuguese Kale and,
        130
poultry
    alternatives to, 67
    avoiding, 5, 58
    chicken
        cancer risk and, 25
        cholesterol in, 76
        fat in, 3–5, *4*, 76, 88
        fiber in, lack of, 9
        heterocyclic amines
            (HCAs) and, 26, 78
    fiber in, lack of, 10, 11
    food safety and, 76
pregnancy, 1, 79
Preventive Medicine Research
    Institute, 54
progesterone-receptor-negative
    tumors, 49
prostate cancer
    calcium as risk to, 18–19, 71
    exercise and, 54, 55
    foods' role in survival of,
        53–56
    low-fat diet's role in, 3, 4
    milk consumption's role in,
        17, 18–20
    soy consumption's effect on,
        81
    studies, 53–56
    tomato products to protect
        against, 31
prostate-specific antigen (PSA),
    54, 55
protein in plant foods. *See also*
    animal

fats/products/protein;
    high-protein diets
    about, 79, 86–88
    amounts of
        American Dietetic Associ-
            ation's guidelines, 27
        for North Americans, 79
        per day/recommended, 7,
            58
        specific, *87*
        variety of, *85*, 87
    chickpeas as source of, 46
    in children's diet, 71
    combining/complementing,
        87
    fat and, 44, 88
    healthfulness of, ix, 26–27
    macrobiotic diet and, 78
    as meat replacement, 27
    refried beans as source of,
        27
    soy products as source of,
        81
PSA (prostate-specific antigen),
    54, 55
pudding(s)
    Harvest, 219
    Rice, 221
    Tapioca, 223
pumpkin
    antioxidants in, *36*
    beta-carotene in, *31*
    as ingredient, in dessert
        recipe, 219
    Pie or Custard, 220
    selenium in, *33*
    as soup thickener, 82
    vitamin E in, *33*

Q

Quèbec City (Canada), 53
Quick Bean Burritos, 207
Quick Fiber Check, 11, *12*, 13
quinoa
    Fruited Breakfast, 94
    *Grains and Cauliflower,
        Mashed,* 168
    Pilaf, 198
    rinsing, 94
    Tacos, 208
    toasting, *163*

R

*Radicchio, and Sesame,
    Spinach Salad with
    Orange,* 149
raisins
    in healthy meal planning, 6,
        22, 60, 87

as ingredient, in breakfast recipes, 94, 96, 98
as ingredient, in dessert recipes, 216, 217, 221
as ingredient, in salad recipe, 136
as snack, 82
raspberry(ies)
  antioxidants in, *37*
  as ingredient, in dessert recipe, 214
  as ingredient, in smoothie recipes, 101, 103
  pesticides in, *64*
  Salad Dressing, 151
Ratatouille Sauce, Chunky, 155
raw foods/raw food diets, 5, 79–80
RDA (Recommended Dietary Allowance), 87
recipe recommendations
  breakfast, 60
  breast cancer, 52
  cancer-fighting/immune-boosting, 42
  dairy alternatives and, 22
  desserts, 62
  dinner, 62
  fiber, 14
  lunch, 61
  meat alternatives and, 27
  New Four Food Groups, 6
  prostate cancer, 56
  weight control, 46
Recommended Dietary Allowance (RDA), 87
red bean(s)
  Casserole, 199
  in *Chili, Three Bean,* 132
  cooking, *13*
  Wraps, 209
red bell pepper(s)
  antioxidants in, *36*
  Hummus, Roasted, 113
  as ingredient, in grain side dish recipes, 166, 167, 170
  as ingredient, in main dish recipes, 188, 194, 201
  as ingredient, in salad recipes
    Asian Fusion, 135
    Bean, Easy, 140
    Bean, Southwest, 147
    Bulgur and Orange, 137
    Citrus Basil, 138
    Fiesta, 141
  as ingredient, in stew recipes, 125, 131

vitamin C in, *34*
red blood cells, 38
refried beans
  in *Burritos, Quick Beans,* 207
  as fiber source, 15
  in healthy meal planning, 46, 61, 62
  as meat replacement, 27
  in *Tostadas, Ten-Minute,* 211
refrigerated items, 66
restaurant dining, 68
retinoic acid, 50
rice. *See also* brown rice; rice cheese; rice milk
  in African/Asian diets, 1, 5, 53
  in low-carbohydrate, high-protein diets, 44
  white, 6, 10, 11, 16
  wild, 66
rice cheese, 64
rice milk
  as alternative
    for cow's milk, viii, 22, 67
    for soy products, 63
    trying, 23
  calcium in
    amount of, *21*
    for children, 72
    as healthy source, 20, 22, 58, 71
  in healthy meal planning, 46, 59
  as ingredient, in breakfast recipe, 94
  as ingredient, in smoothie recipe, 102
  as ingredient, in soup recipe, 129
  in New Four Food Groups, 59
  shakes from, for weight control, 83
  shopping for, 66
  vitamin B$_{12}$ in, 72
roasted foods
  Red Pepper Hummus, 113
  Sweet Potato Wedges, 114
  Vegetables, Sure-Fire, 182
romaine lettuce
  as ingredient, in burrito recipe, 210
  Wraps, Chickpea Salad, 205
Root Soup, Creamy, 123
rutabaga(s)
  calcium in, *21*

as cruciferous vegetable, *34*
  in healthy meal planning, 41
  as ingredient, in side dish recipe, 182
  as ingredient, in soup recipe, 123
  Mashed Potatoes, 179

S
safflower oil, 75
salad(s)
  Asian Fusion, 135
  Bean, Easy, 140
  Bean, Southwest, 147
  Beet, Hot or Cold, 143
  Broccoli, 136
  Bulgur and Orange, 137
  Citrus Basil, 138
  Cucumber, Mango, and Spinach, 139
  fiber from juicing in, 77
  Fiesta, 141
  flaxseed oil added to, 75
  for healthy weight, 46
  Hoppin' John, 142
  Lentil and Bulgur, 144
  Potato, 145
  Romaine Wraps, Chickpea, 205
  sample lunch ideas, 60
  shopping for, 66
  of *Spicy Greens with Fruit and Pine Nuts,* 146
  Spinach, with Citrus Fruit, 148
  Spinach, with Orange, Radicchio, and Sesame, 149
  Tomato, Cucumber, and Basil, 150
  vegetables in, 82
salad dressing(s)
  avoiding, 5
  Balsamic Vinaigrette, 152
  Creamy Dill, 153
  fiber in, 86
  low-fat vegan, 58
  Piquant, 152
  Raspberry, 151
salsa(s)
  Colorful Corn, 108
  Mango, 111
salt (sodium)
  about, 80
  in American diet, 81
  calcium affected by, 22, 71, 72
  cancer risk and, 80
  canned foods and, 13, *14,* 22, 66

sandwiches/burgers/wraps
  Burgers, Chickpea, 204
  Burritos, Quick Bean, 207
  Portobello Mushrooms, Pan-Seared, 206
  sample lunch ideas, 60–61
  Sandwich, Eggless Salad, 203
  Tacos, Quinoa, 208
  Tacos, Soft-Shell, 210
  Tostadas, Ten-Minute, 211
  Wraps, Chickpea Salad Romaine, 205
  Wraps, Red Bean, 209
saturated fat. *See under* fat (dietary)
sauce(s)
  Gravy, Mushroom, 156
  Gravy, Simple Brown, 157
  Marinara, Simple, 156
  Ratatouille, Chunky, 155
  Spaghetti Squash with, 180
  White, Basic, 157
  Sauté, Tempeh Broccoli, 201
  Scramble, Breakfast, 93
  Seasoning Mix, Italian/Mexican/Indian, 183
sea vegetables, 72
seeds. *See also* specific types of
  antioxidants in, *38*
  avoiding/limiting, 5, 46, 58
  beta-carotene in, *38*
  calcium in, *21*
  limiting, 46
  prostate cancer study and, 55
  selenium in, *38*
  vitamin C in, *38*
  vitamin E and, 32, *38*
  for weight gain, 83
seitan
  Buckwheat Pasta with, 189
  as ingredient, in main dish recipes, 194, 200
  as meat replacement, 27, 67
  in New Four Food Groups, 59
  protein in, 58
  serving sizes, *63*
  Stew, Latin, 125
selenium
  about, 32–33
  in beans and legumes, 37
  in fruits, 37
  in grains/grain products, 36
  in healthy meal planning, 41
  minimum daily target, *35*
  in nuts/seeds/oils, 38
  sources of, *33*
  in vegetables, 36

serving sizes
  antioxidants and, *36, 37, 38*
  beta-carotene and, *31*
  of higher-protein plant
    foods, *87*
  lycopene and, *32*
  in New Four Food Groups,
    5, 59
Sesame Salt, Broccoli or Cauli-
  flower with, 174
sesame seeds
  calcium in, *21*
  as ingredient, in appetizer
    recipe, *116*
  as ingredient, in burger
    recipe, *204*
  as ingredient, in main dish
    recipe, *200*
  as ingredient, in salad
    recipes, *148, 149*
  as ingredient, in side dish
    recipes, *172, 174*
  Spinach Salad with Orange,
    Radicchio, and, 149
Seventh-day Adventists, *25*
sex hormone-binding globulin
  (SHBG), *43, 53*
Shanghai (China), *47*
SHBG (sex hormone-binding
  globulin), *43, 53*
Shiitake Mushrooms, Miso
  Soup with, 128
side dishes
  Black Beans and Tomatoes,
    Spicy, 181
  Broccoli or Cauliflower with
    Sesame Salt, 174
  Brown Rice with Black
    Beans, 166
  Bulgur, Chinese Fried, 167
  Calabacitas, 175
  Coleslaw, Asian Persuasion,
    172
  Collard Greens with
    Almonds, 176
  Grains and Cauliflower,
    Mashed, 168
  Kale, Braised, 173
  Pilaf, Brown Rice, 165
  Pilaf, Rice and Carrot, 169
  Pilaf, Tex-Mex Bulgur, 170
  Plantains, Grilled, 177
  Potatoes, Garlic Mashed, 177
  Potatoes, Parsnip Mashed,
    178
  Potatoes, Rutabaga Mashed,
    179
  seasoning mix recipes for,
    183

Spaghetti Squash with Sauce,
  180
Vegetables, Sure-Fire
  Roasted, 182
Yams and Collards, Zippy,
  184
silken tofu. *See under* tofu
simple carbohydrates, *85*
Simple Marinara Sauce, 156
simple sugars, *82*
16 a-hydroxyestrone, *35*
smoking (tobacco)
  by Asians, *81*
  beta-carotene and, *31*
  caffeine and, *69*
  calcium affected by, *22, 71*
  cancer risk and, *vii, 77*
  Seventh-day Adventists and,
    25
smoothie(s)
  Berry-Banana, Mixed, 102
  Blueberry, 100
  Green Goodie, 101
  Green Tea, 103
  Orange Julius, 103
  Strawberry, 104
  Tropical Freeze, 102
snacks
  calcium-rich, *22*
  fruit as, *82*
  sample ideas/suggestions, *62,*
    65
  Soybean, (Edamame), 115
  for weight gain, *83*
snow peas, as ingredient, in
  salad recipe, *135*
soba noodle recipe *(Buckwheat*
  Pasta with Seitan), 189
soda, *11, 82*
sodium. *See* salt (sodium)
Soft-Shell Tacos, 210
soup(s)
  Broccoli, Cream of, 122
  fiber added to, *77*
  instant, *65*
  Kale and Potato, Portuguese,
    130
  Lentil and Brown Rice,
    127
  miso, *80*
    with Shiitake Mushrooms,
      128
  Mushroom Barley, 129
  Root, Creamy, 123
  sample ideas, *60, 62*
  Sweet Potato, Curried, 124
  thickeners for, *82*
  Tomato, with White Beans,
    133

sour cream alternatives/
  substitutes, *23, 67*
Southwest Bean Salad, 147
soybean(s)
  alpha-linoleic acid in, *75*
  antioxidants in, *37*
  cooking, *13*
  fat in, *81*
  in New Four Food Groups,
    59
  omega-3 fatty acids in, *81, 88*
  Snacks (Edamame), 115
soymilk
  as alternative/substitute, *viii,*
    22, 67
  in Asian diet, *81*
  calcium in
    as alternative, *22*
    amount of, *21*
    as healthful source, *20,*
      58, 71, 72
  in New Four Food Groups,
    59
  protein in, *87*
  shakes from, for weight con-
    trol, *83*
  shopping for, *66*
  vitamin B_{12} in, *71–72, 82*
  zinc in, *39*
soy/soy products. *See also* specific types of
  in Asian diet, *81*
  avoiding/limiting, *46, 63*
  fat in, *81*
  fiber in, *81*
  isoflavones in, *81*
  as meat replacement, *27*
  phytoestrogens in, *80, 81*
  processing, *81*
  prostate cancer study and, *55*
soy yogurt, *64, 66, 84*
Spaghetti Squash with Sauce,
  180
Spicy Black Beans and Toma-
  toes, 181
Spicy Greens with Fruit and
  Pine Nuts, Salad of, 146
spinach
  antioxidants in, *36*
  calcium in, *21*
  Dip, Creamy, 109
  as ingredient, in appetizer
    recipes, *116, 118*
  as ingredient, in main dish
    recipes, *191, 193*
  as ingredient, in soup recipe,
    123
  in New Four Food Groups,
    59

  pesticides in, *64*
  in salads, *82*
  Salad with Citrus Fruit, 148
  Salad with Orange, Radic-
    chio, and Sesame, 149
  shopping for, *66*
  Stuffing, Potato Boats with,
    112
  vitamins in, *82*
spirulina
  as ingredient, in smoothie
    recipe, *101*
  vitamin B_{12} in, lack of, *72*
Spread with Sun-Dried Toma-
  toes, White Bean, 119
squash, *59. See also* specific
  types of
stainless steel cookware, *73*
starches, *85*
State University of New York,
  3, 48
stew(s)
  Lentil Artichoke, 126
  Seitan, Latin, 125
  Sweet-and-Sour Vegetable,
    131
  thickeners for, *82*
stir-fry(ies)
  Easy, 190
  fiber from juicing in, *77*
  in healthy meal planning, *x,*
    46, 68
  Sweet-and-Sour, 200
stomach cancer, *35, 80*
strawberry(ies)
  anthocyanins in, *32*
  antioxidants in, *37*
  fiber in, for healthy weight,
    46
  as ingredient, in dessert
    recipes, *214, 222*
  in New Four Food Groups,
    59
  nutrients in, *63*
  pesticides in, *64*
  Smoothie, 104
  vitamin C in, *34*
Stroganoff over Fettuccine,
  Mushroom, 194
stroke, *75, 88*
Stuffed Mushrooms, 116
Stuffing, Potato Boats with
  Spinach, 112
substitutions in recipes, *67, 67,*
  89
sugar, *17, 19, 82, 87*
sugar snap peas, as ingredient,
  in salad recipe, *138*
sulforaphane, *34*

Summer Fruit Compote, 222
Sun-Dried Tomatoes, White Bean Spread with, 119
sunflower oil, 75
sunflower seeds, *33, 38,* 148
sunlight, for vitamin D, 70, 72
supplements, 77, 82. *See also* specific types of
Sweden, 49, 53, *53*
Sweet-and-Sour Stir-Fry, 200
Sweet-and-Sour Vegetable Stew, 131
sweet potato(es)
    antioxidants in, *36*
    cooking's effect on, 73
    as ingredient, in side dish recipe, 182
    as ingredient, in soup recipe, 123
    in meal planning, 61
    Muffins, 98
    in New Four Food Groups, 59
    Soup, Curried, 124
    Wedges, Roasted, 114
Swiss chard, 42, 61, 71

T
Tacos, Quinoa, 208
Tacos, Soft-Shell, 210
tamoxifen, 2
tangerine, as ingredient, in salad recipe, 146
Tapioca Pudding, 23
taste bud memory, 57
tea, 58, 83
Teflon cookware, 73
tempeh
    Broccoli Sauté, 201
    in New Four Food Groups, 59
    phytoestrogens in, 80
    protein in, 87
    serving sizes, 63
    shopping for, 66
    as substitute, 67
    zinc in, *39*
temperature of foods, 76
Ten-Minute Tostadas, 211
testosterone
    cancer risk and, *1, 2, 18, 55*
    reducing, 4, 9, 53
    SHBG's and, 43
Texas Caviar, 117
Tex-Mex Bulgur Pilaf, 170
textured vegetable protein, 87
Thai food, 68
3-3-3 dietary plan, x
Three Bean Chili, 132

three-day dietary record, 6–7
three-week break, *57, 57–58,* 77
tobacco. *See* smoking (tobacco)
tofu
    antioxidants in, 37
    in Asian diet, 81
    Baked, 186
    calcium in, *21*
    firming up, *186*
    French Toast, 95
    as ingredient, in dessert recipe, 215
    as ingredient, in main dish recipe, 193
    as ingredient, in salad dressing recipe, 153
    as ingredient, in sandwich recipe, 203
    as ingredient, in soup recipe, 128
    in New Four Food Groups, 59
    phytoestrogens in, 80
    protein in, 58, 79, 87
    Scramble, Breakfast, 93
    serving sizes, 63
    shakes from, for weight control, 83
    shopping for, 66
    silken
        as alternative, 67
        in *Dressing, Creamy Dill,* 153
        in *Mousse, Chocolate, or Chocolate Mousse Pie,* 215
        in *Sandwich, Eggless Salad,* 203
        as substitute, 67
tomato(es)
    antioxidants in, *36*
    carotenoids in, 41
    Cucumber, and Basil Salad, 150
    as ingredient, in appetizer recipe, 117
    as ingredient, in chili recipes, 121, 132
    as ingredient, in main dish recipes
        Curry (Aloo Gobi), Potato and Cauliflower, 197
        Lasagne, Eggplant, 191
        Lasagne, Lazy, 193
        Loaf, No-Meat, 195
        Squash and Pinto Beans, Home-Style, 192

    Stir-Fry, Sweet-and-Sour, 200
    as ingredient, in salad recipes, 141, 142, 144
    as ingredient, in salsa recipes, 108, 111
    as ingredient, in sandwich recipes, 203
    as ingredient, in sauce recipe, 155
    as ingredient, in soup recipe, 130
    as ingredient, in stew recipes, 125, 126, 131
    as ingredient, in taco recipe, 210
    as ingredient, in tostada recipe, 211
    as ingredient, in wrap recipes, 205, 209
    lycopene in
        amount of, *32*
        antioxidants and, *36*
        cancer risk and, 31, *31, 55*
        in healthy meal planning, 41
        as pigment, 31
    Marinara, Simple, 156
    in meal planning, 41
    in New Four Food Groups, 59
    and Olives, Penne with Kale, 196
    in salads, 82
    Soup with White Beans, 133
    Spicy Black Beans and, 181
    vitamins in, 82
    White Bean Spread with Sun-Dried, 119
Toronto (Canada) study, 54
Tortilla Chips, Baked, 106
Tostadas, Ten-Minute, 211
Tropical Freeze, 102
turnip greens
    calcium and, *21, 22,* 58, 70
    as cruciferous vegetable, *34*
turnips, *34,* 41
2-hydroxyestrone, 35

U
ulcerative colitis, 75, 88
underweight control, 83
University of California, 4, 54, 55
University of Illinois Food Science and Human Nutrition Department, 7
University of Massachusetts, 55

USDA National Nutrient Database for Standard Reference, *4, 31, 33*
U.S. Department of Agriculture, *4, 31, 33*

V
Vancouver (Canada) study, 54
vegan diet
    for cancer patients, 83
    children and, 71–72
    cholesterol in, lack of, 40
    fat and, 48
    fiber in, 86
    healthfulness of, 44
    prostate cancer and, 54, 56
    protein and, 79
    raw foods and, 79–80
    soy products and, 81
    studies about, 44, 51–52, 54
    weight loss and, 44, 45, 51–52
    when traveling, 65
vegetable oils
    avoiding/limiting
        in healthy meal planning, 58, 65, 74
        for weight loss, 44, 45
        when dining out, 68
    estrogen affected by, 1
    fat in, 32, 44, 74, 88
    immune system affected by, 40
    substitutes for, 67, 74
    vitamin E and, 32
    in Western diet, 68
vegetable(s)/veggie(s). *See also* specific types of
    alpha-linoleic acid in, 75
    amino acids in, 79
    amount recommended
        Asian pattern, 5
        daily serving, *5, 59, 63,* 77
    antioxidants in, 29, *29, 36,* 40
    beta-carotene in, *36*
    in a Blanket, 118
    breast cancer and, 49–50
    burgers, 58, 59, 64
    calcium and, 20, 72
    calories in, 44
    in children's diet, 71
    Coconut Curry, Any, 187
    complex carbohydrates in, 85
    cooking's effect on, 72–73, 79–80
    fat and, 4, *4,* 44
    fiber and, 10, 82, 86
    for healthy weight, 46

in low-carbohydrate, high-protein diets, 44
as low-fat food, 26
macrobiotic diet and, 78
in meal planning, 41
in New Four Food Groups, 5, *5*
omega-3 fatty acids in, 88
overcooking, 41
pesticides in, *64*
phytochemicals in, 29, *29*
prostate cancer and, 53, 55, 57
protein in, 26–27, 58, 87
Quick Fiber Check and, 11
sample meal ideas, 60–62
selenium in, *36*
shopping for, 66
Stew, Sweet-and-Sour, 131
in *Stir-Fry, Easy,* 190
supplements vs., 82
Sure-Fire Roasted, 182
vitamin C in, 21, 33, *36,* 72
vitamin E in, *36*
washing, 76
vegetarian diet
cancer and, ix, 25, *25,* 26
for children and adolescents, 71–72
cost of, 73, *74*
fat in, lack of, 51–52
fiber in, 51–52, 86
immune system and, 40–41
of Seventh-day Adventists, 25
weight and, 44
Vinaigrette, Balsamic, 152
vitamins
A, 30, 50, 88
B₁₂, 46, 59, 71–72, 82
C
about, 33
in beans and legumes, *37*
breast cancer and, 50
cooking and, 73
in fruits, *37*
immune system and, ix, 39
iron and, 72
lack of, in dairy products, 77
lack of, in meat, 26
minimum daily target, 35
in nuts/oils/seeds, *38*
sources of, *34*
in vegetables, *36*
in whole grains, *36*
D
calcium and, viii, 18, 19, 20

daily exposure recommended, 70, 72
dietary fat aiding in metabolism of, 88
E
about, 32–33
in barley, 41
in beans and legumes, *37,* 41
in blueberries, 41
breast cancer and, 50
dietary fat aiding in metabolism of, 88
in fruits, *37*
immune system and, 39
minimum daily target, 35
in nuts/oils/seeds, *38*
sources of, *33*
in vegetables, *36*
in whole grains, *36*
K, 88

W
walnuts
alpha-linoleic acid in, 75
antioxidants in, *38*
as ingredient, in breakfast recipe, 91
as ingredient, in main dish recipe, 195
omega-3 fatty acids in, 88
washing hands, 76
water, 11
water chestnuts, as ingredient, in grain side dish recipe, 167
watercress, 41
watermelon
antioxidants in, *37*
lycopene in, 31, *32,* 42, 55
Weaver, C. M., *21*
Wedges, Roasted Sweet Potato, 114
weight
breast cancer and, 40, 43, 47–48, 51
controlling, 43–44, 83–84
fatty foods affecting, 40
gain, after cancer diagnosis, 48
healthy, ix, 43–46
risky diets and, 44–45
studies, 43, 47
sugar's effect on, 82
vegetarian diet's effect on, 40
Western (North American) diet
Asian/African diets vs., 1
breast cancer and, 47, *47*

cancer rate and, 17, *17*
drinking milk in, 17
fat in, 48, 49
fiber in, 13
oil in, 68
protein in, 79
wheat germ, *36, 39, 75,* 88
wheat noodles, 88
wheat protein, 27
WHEL (Women's Healthy Eating and Living) study, 50–51
white bean(s)
antioxidants in, *37*
cooking, *13*
as ingredient, in main dish recipe, 194
as ingredient, in salad recipe, 135
as replacement, 67
Spread with Sun-Dried Tomatoes, 119
Tomato Soup with, 133
white blood cells, 38, 40
white grape juice, as ingredient, in dessert recipe, 222
White Sauce, Basic, 157
whole foods, 56, 77
whole grains. *See also* specific types of
amino acids in, 79
amount recommended, 5, *5,* 59, 63
antioxidants in, *36*
as bean accompaniment, 16
beta-carotene in, *36*
calories in, 44
as cancer fighter, 38
in children's diet, 71
complex carbohydrates in, 85
cooking, *15*
digestion and, 11
fat and, 4, *4,* 44
fiber and, 10, 46, 82
as low-fat food, 26
macrobiotic diet and, 78
Mashed, and Cauliflower, 168
in meal planning, 61
in New Four Food Groups, 5, *5*
omega-3 fatty acids in, 88
phytochemicals in, 38
prostate cancer and, 55, 57
protein in, 26–27, 58, 87
Quick Fiber Check and, 11
sample meal ideas, 59–62
selenium in, 33, *33,* 36

serving sizes, 59, *63*
shopping for, 66
supplements vs., 82
toasting, *163*
vitamin C in, *36*
vitamin E in, *33, 36*
whole wheat bread, 36
WINS (Women's Intervention Nutrition Study), 48
winter squash
as ingredient, in side dish recipe, 182
as soup thickener, 82
Women's Health Initiative study, 2, 49
Women's Healthy Eating and Living (WHEL) study, 50–51
Women's Intervention Nutrition Study (WINS), 48
World Cancer Research Fund, 70
World Health Organization, 75
World War II, 10
wraps. *See* sandwiches/burgers/wraps

Y
yam(s)
antioxidants in, *36*
beta-carotene in, 30, *31*
and Collards, Zippy, 184
Festive Fruited, 216
as ingredient, in stew recipe, 131
shopping for, 66
yellow bell pepper
as ingredient, in main dish recipe, 188
as ingredient, in salad recipe, 141
yellow squash
as ingredient, in side dish recipe, 182
in *Squash and Pinto Beans, Home-Style,* 192
yogurt (dairy), viii, 9, 19, 23

Z
zinc, ix, 39, *39*
Zippy Yams and Collards, 184
zucchini
as ingredient, in breakfast recipe, 92
as ingredient, in side dish recipes, 175, 182
in *Squash and Pinto Beans, Home-Style,* 192

BOOK PUBLISHING COMPANY

since 1974—books that educate, inspire, and empower

To find your favorite vegetarian and alternative health books online, visit:
www.healthy-eating.com

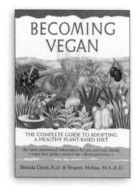

Becoming Vegan
Brenda Davis, RD
& Vesanto Melina, MS, RD
978-1-57067-103-6 $19.95

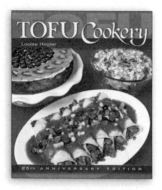

Tofu Cookery
25th Anniversary Edition
Louise Hagler
978-1-57067-220-0 $21.95

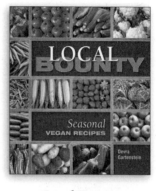

Local Bounty
Devra Gartenstein
978-1-57067-219-4 $17.95

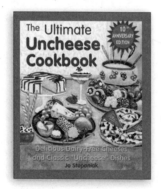

The Ultimate Uncheese
Cookbook
Jo Stepaniak
978-1-57067-151-7 $18.95

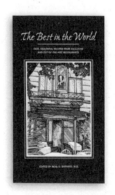

The Best in the World
Edited by Neal D. Barnard, MD
978-0-9664081-0-2 $11.95

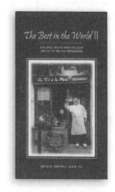

The Best in the World II
Edited by Jennifer L. Keller, RD
& Neal D. Barnard, MD
978-0-9664081-3-3 $11.95

Purchase these health titles and cookbooks from your local bookstore
or natural food store, or you can buy them directly from:

Book Publishing Company • P.O. Box 99 • Summertown, TN 38483
1-800-695-2241

Please include $3.95 per book for shipping and handling.